COGNITIVE BEHAVIORAL THERAPY FOR ANXIETY

Easy Guide to Retraining Your Brain. Learn the Ultimate Techniques to Overcome Anxiety, Stress, Depression, Anger, and Panic Attack. Improve Your Social Skills

© **Copyright 2020 - All rights reserved.**

The content contained within this book may not be reproduced, duplicated or transmitted without direct written permission from the author or the publisher.

Under no circumstances will any blame or legal responsibility be held against the publisher, or author, for any damages, reparation, or monetary loss due to the information contained within this book. Either directly or indirectly.

Legal Notice:

This book is copyright protected. This book is only for personal use. You cannot amend, distribute, sell, use, quote or paraphrase any part, or the content within this book, without the consent of the author or publisher.

Disclaimer Notice:

Please note the information contained within this document is for educational and entertainment purposes only. All effort has been executed to present accurate, up to date, and reliable, complete information. No warranties of any kind are declared or implied. Readers acknowledge that the author is not engaging in the rendering of legal, financial, medical or professional advice. The content within this book has been derived from various sources. Please consult a licensed professional before attempting any techniques outlined in this book.

By reading this document, the reader agrees that under no circumstances is the author responsible for any losses, direct or indirect, which are incurred as a result of the use of information contained within this document, including, but not limited to, errors, omissions, or inaccuracies.

TABLE OF CONTENTS

Introduction 1
Chapter 1: Using Cbt 17
Chapter 2: Identifying Core Beliefs And Values 25
Chapter 3: Understanding Anxiety And The Anxious Mind 35
Chapter 4: Tackling Anxiety, Negativity, And Stress 45
Chapter 5: Triumph Over Anger And Depression 59
Chapter 6: Essential Cognitive Behavior Therapy Techniques 73
Chapter 7: Cognitive Behavioral Treatments For Anxiety 87
Chapter 8: Cognitive Behavioral Treatments For Depression 91
Chapter 9: Cognitive Distortion 95
Chapter 10: Use The Right Kind Of Exercise 109
Chapter 11: You Are Your Own Cure 119
Chapter 12: Maintaining Positive Mindfulness 131
Conclusion 159

INTRODUCTION

You may have heard about Cognitive Behavioral Therapy, the treatment plan that is helping people overcome various mental illnesses. This treatment method has been more successful around the world, and more people are turning to it. If you have been considering to pursue this treatment, it is essential first to understand what you are getting into.

What is CBT?

Cognitive Behavioral Therapy is a type of psychotherapy. It is founded on the perception that most mental illnesses come about as a result of cognitive distortions. Thus, by pointing out these cognitive distortions and adopting helpful beliefs, the patient can overcome their mental illness. Unlike medicine, where it's just about swallowing pills and expecting results, Cognitive Behavioral Therapy requires the full participation of both the patient and the practitioner. Cognitive Behavioral Therapy involves various steps and procedures that must be followed over time. Strict adherence to these steps and procedures always gives positive results. Most Cognitive Behavioral Therapy techniques can be practiced in day-to-day life, which means there is no limit to your improvement. Cognitive Behavioral Therapy takes on a holistic healing philosophy, and what's more, you get to understand how your brain perceives various things and people. In other words, Cognitive Behavioral Therapy helps you increase your self-awareness.

Did you know the number one cause of marital problems is poor communication? And when we talk about poor communication, we don't mean to say that partners have refused to speak to each other. They are talking to each other. But the problem is that each one of them gets a different message rather than what is intended. There are very many psychological factors that stop partners from understanding each other clearly. The importance of Cognitive Behavioral Therapy is that it draws attention to some of these factors that ultimately sabotage a relationship.

Cognitive Behavioral Therapy helps treat various conditions such as phobias, anxiety, major depressive disorder, dissociative disorder, personality disorders, self-esteem, and self-image issues.

Cognitive Behavioral Therapy helps the patient understand most of their thought processes and see the connection between how they think and how they act. Since this treatment plan came into being, a lot of studies have been made to see its effectiveness, and so far, this treatment plan is beneficial. Cognitive Behavioral Therapy posts even better results than people who are on medication.

Is CBT for me?

. In actual fact, the success of Cognitive Behavioral Therapy depends on the patient's effort. Thus, before you decide to follow this treatment plan, you must be ready to commit to the procedures, else you may end up wasting both your time and money.

What takes place during Cognitive Behavioral Therapy sessions & how long does it last?

At the start, the practitioner will find a way of ensuring that you both connect. Most practitioners have worked on their personalities, and they know how to handle different kinds of people. So, it is not uncommon for a practitioner to want to know about their patient's background. This helps them understand their patients even more. The practitioner opens up about the realities of Cognitive Behavioral Therapy. The patient needs to be aware of the various struggles that they will run into.

The practitioner gets to ask about the problem that is dogging their patients. And the patient must try to be as forthcoming as possible. Some people are tempted to hold back parts that they feel ashamed of, but this is not a smart move; you must let it all out. Then the practitioner offers the patient various steps and procedures that are aimed at identifying your cognitive distortions. The patient must adhere to these steps and procedures.

The amount of time it takes to achieve positive results with Cognitive Behavioral Therapy is dependent on the efforts of both the practitioner and the patient, and also the kind of problem being dealt with. But in a general sense, Cognitive Behavioral Therapy is more time-efficient than various other treatment methods. For instance, if you swallowed pills to become euphoric and numb yourself from feelings of low self-esteem, you might have to take those pills forever. But when it comes to Cognitive Behavioral Therapy, it is a matter of establishing the root cause of your self-esteem issues, and then developing new positive beliefs about yourself, and applying these principles into your daily life, and the self-esteem issue is gone.

Using Cognitive Behavioral Therapy techniques beyond the course

One of the benefits of Cognitive Behavioral Therapy is the fact that you can continue practicing these steps way after your class. A skilled practitioner will give you knowledge. And this knowledge is what keeps you going. You will find that various stages won't require any spending of money. It is up to you to just find the time. So, by incorporating these Cognitive Behavioral Therapy steps into your life, you solidify the effectiveness of this treatment plan. There are various resources, such as books, magazines, and online portals, to help you along the way.

Does science support CBT? Is it successful?

Some people might want to find out whether Cognitive Behavioral Therapy is backed by science. This is a very legitimate concern, considering that most people are a victim to pseudo-scientific disciplines. Scientists have analyzed the effectiveness of Cognitive Behavioral Therapy. They have studied how patients that go through the entire course of Cognitive Behavioral Therapy fare against similar patients who have undergone other forms of treatment. They found out that patients who have undergone Cognitive Behavioral Therapy tend to recover fully simply because the results are lasting. But for patients who, e.g., Take medicine, they might relapse into their previous mental state, which is basically back to step one.

During a CBT course, these are some of the things that you will learn:

•**Identify problems more clearly:** CBT helps you have a clearer picture of what's behind your questions. Talk therapy is designed to get to the root of the problem.

•**Develop an awareness of automatic thoughts**: your automatic thoughts are responsible for your negative behaviors and actions. CBT helps you understand your automatic thoughts when they come up.

•**Challenge underlying assumptions that may be wrong**: negative thoughts and twisted perceptions can stem from inaccurate presumptions.

CBT helps you uncover the incorrect assumptions you may hold.

•**Distinguish between facts and irrational thoughts**: some complications come about as a result of holding onto irrational thoughts for the longest time. CBT helps you identify what's factual and get rid of the irrational beliefs that have held you as a hostage as well as given you bad traits.

•**Understand how past experiences can affect present experiences**: for most people who struggle with mental health issues, particularly depression, their past is to blame. Something traumatic went down in the past that triggered their depression. CBT helps them identify what these past problems are and get over them. The healing process starts once they have overcome their terrible past experiences.

•**Stop fearing the worst**: most people develop mental illnesses that are anchored on their fear for the worst. For instance, if you tend to worry about what would happen if you are alone in a dark room, CBT helps you understand that nothing would happen at all, and your fear is imagined.

- **See a situation from a different perspective:** one of the problems that people have when it comes to mental illnesses is an inability to have various aspects to the same thing. Most negative thought patterns can be overcome when you start perceiving life from more than one angle. It stimulates your creativity and helps you overcome your present challenge.

- **Better understand other peoples' actions and motivations:** we don't live in a vacuum. We live in a space inhabited by other people. Their efforts are bound to influence our lives, whether we like it or not. Thus, we had better understand other peoples' actions and motivations. If we know what motivates them, we are in a better position to take self-preserving decisions and not falling prey to them.

- **Develop a more positive way of thinking and seeing situations:** the value of keeping a positive mind in the face of trouble cannot be overstated. It makes all the difference. CBT helps people develop a positive mindset and face their challenges without falling into vices and other harmful habits.

- **Become more aware of their mood**: if you are battling mental illnesses, you are likely to experience terrible feelings most of the time. CBT helps you uncover the relationship between your thoughts, actions, and beliefs. If you engage in harmful activities, you have a high likelihood of experiencing low moods.

•**Establish attainable goals:** at the end of the day, everyone wants to see their dreams come true. The problem is that some of these dreams are more life delusions. If you set a goal that has no chance of ever coming to life, you set yourself up for failure. CBT helps you stay grounded and have the presence of mind required to craft attainable goals.

•**Avoid generalizations and all-or-nothing thinking:** we shouldn't think in absolute terms. There are certainly gray areas. By embracing CBT, we get to understand the value of paying attention to the gray areas instead of an all-or-nothing mindset.

•**Stop blaming yourself:** some people shift blame to themselves for things that were totally beyond their control. This makes it hard for them to overcome the problem. Through CBT, they can understand the value of objectivity and not just burdening themselves with unwarranted blame.

- **Focus on the present:** CBT might help you understand your past and prepare for the future, but the main emphasis is the present. CBT techniques are aimed at working with whatever that's going on at present. Thus, CBT provides a very accurate remedy for your troubles.

- **Face your fears:** if you have been battling concerns, you might have developed several negative thinking patterns, and twisted perception of reality, that have no doubt gifted you a mental illness such as paranoia or phobias. CBT helps you face your fears and emerge triumphantly.

How CBT works?

Your actions are influenced by your thoughts, feelings, and physical sensations. When you give room to negative thoughts, you end up trapped in a cycle of degenerative behaviors and actions. CBT helps you break down a problem into small bits so that you can deal with it far easier. It allows you to change these negative patterns to improve how you feel. Unlike other treatment models that focus on past issues, CBT focuses on what's troubling you at present, promoting appropriate thoughts, behaviors, and habits.

Problems are broken down into five main groups:

- Physical feelings
- Situations
- Actions
- Thoughts
- Emotions

These five areas are interconnected. For instance, your thoughts about a specific location might affect your feelings, as well as the response that you are going to give. CBT is different from other psychotherapies in the following aspects:

- **It's pragmatic**: specific problems are identified, and work begins in solving them.

- **Highly structured:** the therapist and the patient identify particular challenges and set goals as a way of finding a solution.

- **Focused on the present**: CBT focuses on what your thoughts, emotions, and habits are like at present as opposed to focusing on your past.

- **Collaborative:** the success of this talking therapy is, in a significant sense, dependent upon the relationship between the therapist and the patient. The two must work together to find a lasting solution.

There are convenient and inconvenient ways of approaching a problem, depending on your thought system. For example, if your marriage partner deserts you and files for divorce, you might think that you are a failure, and consider yourself unworthy of finding love again. This line of thought could make you hopeless and lonely, turning you into a hermit that detests people and trapped in a vicious cycle of negativity, you feel bad about yourself and self-sabotage against ever being in a meaningful relationship.

On the other side, you could make peace with the fact that divorce is not the end of your love life. Many people get past it and live to their full potential. Developing optimism for the future will influence your habits and actions. You will start going out more, taking up different activities, and eventually, you'll run into someone that your heart beats for.

The above example is a perfect illustration of how your thoughts, feelings, and physical sensations can hold you in a cycle of negativity, and even create new situations that worsen how you feel about yourself. It shows that if you want to turn your life around, you must begin by exploring your mental constitution, and commit to altering your thoughts and feelings.

CBT seeks to put an end to such negative cycles, by exposing the associated thoughts and emotions and empowering you to turn your life around. CBT techniques are designed in such a manner that after a certain point, you don't need a therapist to break the negative cycles, but just your dedication.

CBT Sessions

You can carry out CBT sessions as an individual or a group with a therapist, but if you have some substantial experience, you might not even need a therapist. If you have CBT as an individual or as a group, you'll generally meet with the therapist five to twenty times for weekly or fortnightly sessions, with each session taking about 30 – 60 minutes. The sessions may take place anywhere both of you are comfortable: clinic, outdoor, home.

Cognitive Behavioral Therapy Techniques

These are some of the techniques in CBT used to modify a person's behavioral patterns:

•**Cognitive rehearsal**: the patient starts by calling to mind their traumatic events, and with the help of a therapist, they work toward a solution. The patient has to instill positive thoughts in their mind to strengthen their positive attitude and encourage the development of positive traits. The part about rehearsing positive thoughts requires a bit of imagination.

•**Validity testing**: in this technique, the therapist seeks to test whether the patient's beliefs are valid or invalid. The patient can bring up objective evidence to defend their feelings, but if their argument is weak, then the inaccuracy of their belief is exposed, and they are encouraged to create accurate opinions.

•**Writing a journal**: a patient takes upon themselves to note down the happenings of their life to trace maladaptive behaviors. The patient notes down all the critical things taking place in their life, at the emotional, mental, and physical plane, and together with the therapist, they may review these events to find out the interconnectedness between these areas.

•**Guided discovery**: patients may exhibit negative tendencies when they have a flawed perception of reality. But a therapist would assist them in comprehending their cognitive distortions. Patients become more aware of how they process information. In the end, patients can adopt an accurate perception of reality, and it helps them process information accurately.

•**Modeling:** it is one of the most critical techniques in straightening out a patient. A therapist may perform role-playing exercises from which the patient may draw inspiration to change their behavior. It helps the patient understand the perfect ways of response to various scenarios.

•**Homework**: in this technique, the patient is asked to perform multiple tasks to draw lessons that will impact their mindset and help them modify their behaviors. Some of the functions include reviewing audiotapes, taking notes, and reading articles.

- **Systematic positive reinforcement**: in this technique, a patient is encouraged to bring out more of their positive traits. It's far easier to modify a person's behaviors when their positive characteristics are dominant. Thus, a therapist would identify a patient's positive characteristics, and then reward the patient for every time their positive habits or attitudes are applied.

CHAPTER 1
USING CBT

When you decide that CBT is the best process through which you can defeat your anxiety, you likely want to prepare yourself and learn what to expect. When you think of therapy, you probably assume that there will be a lounge for you to rest upon with a stoic man dressed in all dark colors writing on a clipboard while you speak, or you may assume that you will be looking at blotches on a piece of paper to see where your mind goes first. While those are stereotypical, they could not be further from the truth with CBT. CBT is focused on being active rather than passive and is not interested in interpreting the patterns ink creates on paper. Instead, CBT wants to teach you skills.

What to Expect?

If you engage in CBT in person, you can expect to meet with a therapist that is interested in teaching you directly.

He or she will want to get an idea of what kinds of issues you may be having, as well as how best to help you manage anxiety.

You will likely spend a great deal of time, in the beginning, discussing your symptoms and thoughts, though this is atypical in the future.

With a general assessment of where you fall on the anxiety spectrum and the kind of person you are, the therapist will then begin to tailor a set of skills that he or she believes will be most beneficial to you.

The therapist will choose out skills that will directly help whatever problem you have.

If you have a phobia, for example, you will likely be facing graded exposure. If you have a sincerely believed thought that you are unworthy of love, you are likely to go through some severe cognitive reconstruction.

The methods that work for one person may not work for another, so it is essential to get that general baseline at the beginning of the process.

With the general information figured out, you can expect each of your one-hour sessions to be broken down into a period of time, discussing the last week's homework and progress you have made in your own life. This is the sort of check-in ensuring that you are actually making progress and that you are able to use the skills that are being taught. You will discuss how successful you have been in your attempts to change your mindset, as well as address any concerns that may have come up for you.

From there, you are likely to spend a period of time learning a new skill relevant to your particular case and symptoms. You will practice with the therapist, using all sorts of role-playing, thought experiments, and other kinds of methods to explore the new techniques. As you learn them, you will then be tasked with using them for the next period of time between appointments.

This homework is crucial, and it is meant to give you experience using the techniques being taught in real-time, away from the therapist, and in legitimate settings.

You learn to cope with legitimate stressors using the abilities taught in the therapy, and with every success you have, you experience encouragement and a desire to repeat that success in the future.

As you develop the skills necessary, you will find that you grow more and more skilled at dealing with stress as it comes up. At your next appointment, then, you will discuss your previous week's homework once more to identify strong and weak areas for you.

When you engage in CBT on your own, however, the process is slightly different. Remember, CBT is active and you need to be practicing in order to see any real success and benefit to the process. You are at a disadvantage because you do not have a licensed professional guiding the process and customizing any of the techniques to make them relevant specifically to you. You do not have a bouncing board on which to work out ideas. Instead, you are mostly responsible for the process yourself. You need to figure out how best to cope with your issues, and you need to figure out which techniques are more or less effective than others are. Without the therapist or professional to guide you, you also have no one keeping you accountable for your progress. You are stuck figuring out the process on your own, with no help, and for some people, that is intimidating mainly.

It can, of course, be done, if you are willing to motivate yourself, but many people may find the process daunting.

Remember, it is entirely acceptable for you to decide halfway through the process that you would rather have a therapist there to guide you.

It is also acceptable to feel stuck sometimes and struggle with how to move forward—this is a process, and processes take time.

What you can do is take notes on what works for you and read plenty of different books on the subject, looking for a wide range of techniques that will benefit you. You can also look for worksheets and guides online to help you as well if you feel like you need the added support. You can even find groups of people to talk to online that are going through similar processes.

Remember, the essential part, regardless of whether you are engaging in CBT yourself or with a therapist, is to remain diligent and dedicated. It will take practice to see desired results, but if you are willing to put in the effort, you will not be disappointed.

How it Helps

CBT helps because it teaches you how best to cope with problems. It does not seek to identify and solve one specific problem, but rather, give you the tools necessary to fix any problem. It is the difference between someone walking over and handing a hungry person a fish versus giving the hungry person a fishing pole and teaching him how to catch his own food. While giving the fish helps, the individual is still going to run into issues with hunger down the road. When you teach him how to fish, however, and give him the tools necessary to do so, you ensure that he is able always to catch whatever it is he needs to maintain that he never goes hungry again.

Psychotherapy versus CBT :

In many other forms of psychotherapy, the therapist will guide you to an answer for that one particular issue you are there for. However, you are likely to struggle again in the future, you are going to run into situations in which you struggle to cope, and you fall back into old behavioral patterns. CBT knows that bad things happen to everyone, and sometimes everyone needs to spend time coping with something. CBT knows that there will be future traumas, and because of that, CBT encourages you to develop skills necessary in the future. You not only learn how to solve your current problem, you learn how to solve the future ones as well. In doing so, you are able to repeatedly engage in any productive behavior necessary to problem-solving without needing repeated therapy. If you realize that you are now anxious about something else, you can engage in the coping mechanisms you learned in CBT. When someone has gone through talk therapy or relied on medication, on the other hand, the individual is likely to need to go back to therapy or get back on medication to see the same relief that worked before.

CHAPTER 2
IDENTIFYING CORE BELIEFS AND VALUES

One of the first steps you engage in when you begin the process of CBT is learning how to identify core beliefs and values. When you are able to do that, you are able to begin the process of identifying problematic thoughts. When you want to identify a core value, you are essentially signing yourself up to delve deep into your mind, diving into your unconscious thoughts and feelings in hopes of gaining insight into your situation. These beliefs and values are largely unnoticed in your day-to-day life unless you actively know how to look for them and decide to do so, so most people struggle even to acknowledge them. When you learn to do so, however, you unlock an important skill necessary to understand yourself.

When you learn to identify your core beliefs, you begin to understand your own motivators, learning about the things that make you behave the way you do. This is crucial to this process, which is all about recognizing the cycle between thoughts, feelings, and behaviors. You are essentially learning to identify the thoughts within that cycle so you can learn how to best cope with them.

What are the Core Beliefs and Values?

Core beliefs are automatic thoughts that you have that you believe wholeheartedly are true about yourself. They compose the way you think of yourself, influencing everything from how you behave to what you think you deserve in relationships.

They determine whether you put up with abuse or assume that you deserve to be abandoned or rejected. They determine how likely you are to anything, and they occur without you being aware of them.

Your core beliefs exist deep in your unconscious, swaying your behavior without requiring you to use up any important cognitive resources considering things. They decide many of your emotional, instinctive behaviors, and you always default to them. You will always take your core beliefs as factual unless you are given a good enough reason to reject them. Even then, rejecting them can be a long, arduous struggle on its own simply because you do not want to admit that you do not know your own behaviors and personality type. In correcting your core beliefs, you are essentially declaring that you do not know how to judge yourself and that you do not have a good understanding of who you are as a person.

How do Core Beliefs Impact Behavior?

Core beliefs have a major impact on behavior. They are determining factors for much of your own behavioral patterns. When you act upon your core beliefs, you are essentially behaving in ways that you accept to be true inherently. For example, if you have a core belief that says that your family and friends all reject you in the end because you are unworthy of love or affection, you will always approach relationships feeling guarded and tense. You will constantly assume the worst in those around you, which can have a hugely negative impact on your relationships, pushing people away, and of course, as soon as someone chooses to leave the relationship after being treated accordingly, you automatically assume it is to justify your core belief.

This can go even further, with you even contorting what has happened around you into delusional interpretations of what has happened. If your friend legitimately is held up at work, for example, and has to cancel your girls' night out, you may immediately convince yourself that it is, in fact, proof that your friend does not like you. You assume that your friend is intentionally trying to lie to you, and instead of behaving in an understanding manner, you get standoffish and offended before getting upset simply because you assume it was intentionally done to bother you.

Identifying Core Beliefs with CBT

Identifying core beliefs is a relatively simple concept to understand, though the process can cause distress. It is common for people to feel upset or distressed as they parse through their thoughts and feelings simply because they are uncovering some of these distortions that imply that they believe they are not good enough. They are essentially admitting that even they, themselves, believe they are unworthy of care and attention, and in doing so, they have to admit that the one person that should like them, themselves, have low opinions.

When you want to identify a core belief, what you are going to do is approach the situation first with identifying the thought behind an emotion, and then attempt to analyze it until you arrive at a statement about yourself. For example, you may feel anxious about your social interactions, believing that they are largely unhappy because no one legitimately likes you.

You may point to a recent time in which you felt intense sadness and anxiety. That intense feeling is there to tell you that something was wrong there, and you need to pay attention to it to get to the root of the situation. Identify that situation and ask yourself what happened at that moment. You may notice that it coincided with your friend having to skip out on girls' night because she was too busy at work and was forced into mandatory overtime. You felt sad, followed by anxiety, followed by anger.

Now that you have that feeling identified, you should take a moment to understand what those feelings implied about you. You may spend some time reflecting on the situation before finally settling on the fact that feeling upset meant that you felt insecure. That is a good observation, but it is not the end of the thought chain. You must then consider what that means to you. You may ask why you feel so insecure and consider why. The answer may be something along the lines of feeling as though you are unimportant or unwanted in your friends' groups. Again, consider why that matter—you may decide that you feel like people only like you out of pity. One last time, identify why that is relevant to you and what that says about you, and you reach the core belief: You feel unworthy and undeserving of love.

With that core belief identified, you are then ready to move on to other steps in the CBT process. There are, of course, several ways that you could go through this process to identify any core beliefs you hold. For example, you could use journaling to go through that process or decide that you would rather do self-reflection, simply letting your thoughts run loose and dictate where they go on their own.

Journaling

Some people prefer to resort to journaling to understand their thought processes. This is actually quite smart—it enables you to have a relatively easy to follow written record of the thoughts you are tracking, and in developing them, you will be able to understand how you think. This can be essential, especially if you are trying to understand behavioral or thought patterns that you may hold.

When you want to engage in journaling, one of the most important points is ensuring that you have a quiet time in which you can stop and consider what is happening without stress or interruption. You want to be able to entirely focus on your train of thought as you go through this process. Try setting aside the same time every day for a chance to reflect.

Once you sit down to journal, stop, and consider any trains of thought you may have at that particular moment. You want to know exactly what is on your mind and acknowledge it. Then, follow that one train of thought, identifying what it means to you, how it is relevant, and searching for the core belief at the heart of it. As you do this, over time, you will begin to uncover more and more core beliefs about yourself. While this does not necessarily have any structure, it helps to keep each journal entry limited somewhat to a similar theme so you can analyze it to understand how it relates.

Your thought process likely looks something like this in written form:

Notice how the chain is a repeated attempt to identify the meaning of the previous realization all the way down until you arrive at the core belief or thought behind the process. This is important—you are essentially spiraling down the rabbit hole of your thoughts and implications until you reach the truth that you hold.

Self-Reflection

Self-reflection, again, follows a similar pattern. When you are self-reflecting, however, you are going to follow the trains of thought within yourself.

You are not focusing so much on writing down what has occurred so much as pursuing your natural trains of thought. You simply allow your thoughts to go without stopping them, waiting to see where they end up eventually.

This is for those who struggle to journal or write about emotions, or perhaps people who cannot write at that moment, such as if they are driving but would like to get to the core beliefs located at the heart of some pretty negative emotional reactions.

The important part is not so much to get everything written down, but rather to ensure you understand yourself. You need to recognize how you truly feel about yourself, and when you learn to recognize that, you can then begin to cope with it or change it to something effective that you would rather see yourself as. Either way, you develop a useful skill as a result of identifying the core belief.

Remember, no matter the method you choose to identify your core beliefs, you are likely to feel some pretty strong emotions. This is okay and even expected in many situations, and despite the emotions you feel, you need to recognize that you are worth going through the process. It is worth challenging these beliefs despite the fact that doing so can and likely will bring about pain as well. When you are challenging these beliefs, you are essentially challenging yourself as a person, despite the fact that your perception of you may very well be too negative actually to be healthy or maintained, or even accurate to begin with. It is okay to get upset, and it is even okay to cry—understand that the pain says it is working. All healing processes involve pain, but that is okay—the pain says your body and mind are processing the issues you are facing, and in processing them, you are able to better cope in the future.

CHAPTER 3
UNDERSTANDING ANXIETY AND THE ANXIOUS MIND

Historical Treatment of Anxiety

The World Health Organization (WHO) reported that 300 million people worldwide suffer from depression. That is almost 1/5th of the world's population. Depression is also believed to be the No.1 contributing disability in the world. Anxiety disorders ranked sixth. These statistics are sad reading. The US has one of the highest rates of anxiety. With eight people in every 100, suffering anxiety disorders in some form WHO (2017).

Studies are also showing that common mental health disorders occur at a higher rate in the lower-income sectors. Even more disturbing is the fact that anxiety disorders are treatable. Why then are the figures so high? Is it a modern epidemic?

In medieval times treatment consisted of blood leaches and bathing in freezing water. It was a real breakthrough when psychologists such as Sigmund

Freud, started treating sufferers more like patients. Such patients began to undergo the "talking" therapy. It was not until as late as the 1980's that the American Psychiatric Association recognized "anxiety" as a mental health disorder. Before then, anxiety was simply classed as a "woman's problem." Sufferers became stigmatized and labeled as depressives. Women are twice as likely to suffer from anxiety disorders, but such conditions are by no means restricted to females only. Today, anxiety may be treated with medication as well as therapy.

What is Anxiety?

In days gone by, our ancestors risked their lives whenever they hunted live food. Luckily, these skills are no longer needed, but it brings us to how the body reacts when facing danger. This is a time when we instinctively make the decision of "fight, flight, or freeze." It's not a choice brought on by conscious thought. Rather, it is set in motion by the release of chemicals in the part of our brain known as the limbic system. The chemical is cortisol, which is a steroid hormone released through the adrenalin glands. One of the side effects of raised levels of this hormone is anxiety. If you feel this type of anxiety too often, the high levels of cortisol can damage cells in a part of the brain known as the hippocampus. This is an area that helps process memories. Such damage can lead to impaired learning and loss of memory. McAuley et al. (2009)(2a). de Quervain et al. (1998) (2b).

Symptoms of Anxiety

Anxiety is now separated from the condition of depression. Although many who suffer from depression also have anxiety issues. Patients who suffer from depression tend to dwell on the past and feel very negative about themselves and life in general. This is not typical in the case of patients suffering from anxiety. They will worry excessively about the here and now or the future. Their lives are full of "what ifs" in the eventuality of a disaster. Symptoms of anxiety can vary in individuals, but here are a few to look out for:

- Feeling tense for no reason, on edge, and almost nervous.
- The sense of dread and impending doom.
- Unable to sleep because of worry.
- General restlessness and fidgeting, unable to

relax.

- Lack of concentration.
- Irritable for no reason.
- Breaking out in a cold sweat.
- Shaking.
- Feeling nauseous.
- Digestive and intestinal upsets.

Panic attacks can come as a result of feeling one or many of these symptoms. When someone has frequent anxiety attacks, it inevitably leads to ill health. This is because of the cortisol levels remain high too often and for too long. One of cortisol's roles is to increase blood sugars. Unbalanced, and this can result in insulin resistance. In turn, this may lead to late-onset or type 2 diabetes. Hacket et al. (2016) (2c).

In a modern, fast-paced society with access to social media, many people are feeling more and more anxious about the world around us. This can start at an early age. If young people are not diagnosed and treated, their anxiety attacks will follow them into adulthood.

There are also various stages throughout life that can lead to feeling over anxious:

- **Education**

Learning and education should be an enjoyable experience. All too often, children are pressured to meet certain academic targets. Those who don't meet them may very well consider themselves a failure. The burden of being successful lays heavy on the shoulders of young people.

- **Family life.**

This is a worrying time, particularly if you have never had responsibilities. Women are expected to raise families and go out to work at the same time. Such pressures create huge stresses in their daily lives. With the increasing break up of marriages, the pressure of anxiety reflects on both parents, and on the children.

- **Materialism**

People who live in wealthy industrialized countries are bombarded with a heavily commercialized culture. Advertising constantly prompts us to buy the newest and seemingly greatest ever products. Such deviant tactics imply that their goods will improve your life and make you happy. It seems we must keep up with all the latest gadgets to have an attractive home, and wear the latest fashion labels to look good. All were increasing the pressures of life as we attempt to earn more money to keep up.

- **The Anxious Mind**

Whilst it might seem to be stating the obvious, and worry plays a key role in anxiety. People who suffer from anxiety attacks are likely big worriers. Often, the only way a worrier will stop panicking over a specific problem is if they have moved on to a different one. Worry leads to anxiety until the released chemicals mean the person cannot think rationally. At this point, they will jump to conclusions of their own making. Unable to focus on reality because their minds are highly aroused, the problem is no longer solvable. They cannot see any solutions, which then leads deeper into anxiety.

- **Simple Coping Techniques**

For those who experience the build-up of burdening pressures and suffer anxiety attacks, there is help available. We will look at this in more detail later in this book. There are lifestyle changes that can be put into practice, using techniques to nip the anxiety attacks in the bud. A sufferer may find that these techniques are all they need to **alleviate the experience of anxiety. Such as:**

- Discussing your anxiety issues with your doctor. Doctors can prescribe medication to help you initially, and then refer you to a CBT therapist.

- Look at the foods you eat and what you drink. Caffeine and alcohol can both affect anxiety levels negatively. Take the general advice and at the very least, cut down on the intake of foods known to cause such effects.

- Exercise is beneficial, but it doesn't mean you must work-out like crazy at a gym. Go on walks in calm and soothing vistas, if possible. Learn relaxation exercises that you can do sitting at a desk or watching TV, such as breathing exercises and muscle relaxation.

- Try and keep active, so you tire yourself out naturally during the day. That way, sleep will come easier at night.

Stress and anxiety are closely related conditions. Though it is possible to suffer one without suffering the other, for both, you should seek help, but there are many self-help techniques that you can do to ease some of the immediate pressures.

Anxiety can include phobias and is often only triggered in certain circumstances. Stress is more a build-up of worry because there is too much pressure in your life. Something has to give. We will look at ways of helping yourself to cope with anxiety. Many of the coping methods are ways to ease the pressures, are similar to the stress self-help approach. It could be that stress is what has brought on your anxiety in the first place. Deal with one, and the other may ease as well.

Recognizing that you are suffering from anxiety is the first stage. Events such as employment interviews will naturally cause anxious feelings; these are normal. You should not worry about anxiety when associated with common stressful events. Having adrenalin coursing through your system when under such stress is a way your body copes with the situation. When you come out of the interview, the anxiety should lift to be replaced with relief that the stress is over. Of course, you may then stress while you wait for the results but try not to be over-anxious in such situations.

It is when you are anxious over too many things, especially every day and maybe even all day. This is unhealthy as you will be producing those hormones we mentioned earlier, in high amounts. If you find that stress is affecting your everyday life, then it is time to seek help. The stress will mount up, causing triggers to anxiety attacks. Hopefully, you will recognize the dire situation before it gets to that point.

If you have suffered anxiety attacks for over 6 months, this is known as Generalized Anxiety Disorder (GAD).

CHAPTER 4
TACKLING ANXIETY, NEGATIVITY, AND STRESS

Anxiety is a word that is quite common to most people, but funnily enough, not many people can define the word. When you experience a feeling of worry, nervousness, or unease about something, or maybe about the uncertainty of an outcome, then you are anxious.

Anxiety, in itself, is usually a disorder that affects how we feel or behave. This disorder can even cause some physical symptoms. However, if you are facing such impairment, you don't have to live with it. Anxiety is treatable.

The best approach to take with the aim of treating is to take on some therapy sessions. Cognitive Behavioral Therapy (CBT), Psychotherapy, and Exposure Therapy are some of the therapies one may majorly consider. The thing with these therapies is that they will help you in controlling your anxiety levels and even help you conquer your fears.

Treating Anxiety Disorders

Some may ask the question: "Why should I go through some hectic therapy session just to treat the disorder while I can simply buy medication and achieve the same result in the comfort of my house?" That can be an excellent way to tackle it, but the problem is that it is only short term. This is because the medication will just eliminate the physical symptoms, leaving behind the underlying causes of your worries and nervousness.

Research has shown that therapy is an effective method to tackle anxiety. How? It simply gives you the tools to overcome your fear and teaches you how to use them.

Therapies are usually considered long-term by most people. However, this is not the case with CBT-based anxiety therapy. Surprisingly, within the first eight to ten months, many people are usually okay. The length of these therapies is generally measured by the severity of the disorder, and also the type. The different kinds of anxiety disorders include Generalized Anxiety Disorder (GAD), Obsessive-Compulsive Disorder (OCD), Panic Disorder, and many more. It is now also obvious to note that therapy should be tailored to one's specific symptoms. A person suffering from GAD cannot undergo the same therapy session as one suffering from OCD.

As earlier said, various types of anxiety therapies that can be considered are in existence. However, the two leading treatments are Cognitive Behavioral Therapy and Exposure Therapy. These therapies can be used alone or be accompanied by other types of treatment. Another thing to note is that these therapies can be done at an individual level or to a group of people who have the same anxiety problems. We are going to cover the CBT part.

Cognitive Behavioral Therapy for Anxiety

Cognitive Behavioral Therapy primarily works to alleviate both negative cognitions, that is, thoughts and beliefs, and also maladaptive behaviors associated with anxiety. CBT seeks to blend the best parts of behavior and cognitive therapies.

As the name suggests, there are two main components of this therapy: Cognitive Therapy and Behavioral Therapy. Cognitive therapy is the part that involves one's thoughts. This part examines how one's negative thoughts contribute to anxiety.

Behavioral treatment, on the other hand, examines one's behavior and reactions when in situations that trigger anxiety. It is important to note that this type of treatment mainly focuses on our thoughts rather than the events. This is because one's thoughts determine one's feelings. Let's take an event, like that of getting a job somewhere you never thought you would ever be employed. This event can lead to various feelings, which are determined by how you think about the situation. For example:

- The thought that you are fortunate to have landed in such a job will make you feel thrilled and jovial.

- Thinking that you are under-qualified enough for such a high-end job may make you feel undeserving of the opportunity, and this can lead to stress.

The above represents the same situation but two very different feelings that can be achieved by merely how you think.

Generally, for people with anxiety disorders, their decisions are often clouded with negative thoughts that lead to negative emotions of worry, nervousness, or fear. For such people, Cognitive Behavioral Therapy usually comes in handy because it helps them identify and fight these negative thoughts, thereby avoiding negative emotions that cause anxiety.

Thought Challenging in CBT

Thought challenging is a useful technique used in CBT that helps one consider situations from multiple angles, using actual evidence from your life. It involves challenging one's negative thoughts and replacing them with more positive and realistic opinions.

This technique usually involves three steps. Namely:

1. Identifying Negative Thoughts

Anxiety and negative thoughts are a very evil duo that can lead to very severe problems. People with anxiety disorder tend to perceive things or events more seriously than other people. For example, a person who fears dogs will consider touching them as life-threatening. Somebody else will view this as safe as long as he or she approaches the dog in a friendly way. This step can be tough to take because identifying one's fear is not that simple.

This is the only sure way to determine your fear.

2. Challenging Negative Thoughts

Once the fears and the negative thoughts have been identified, the next thing is to test these thoughts. What does this mean? It basically means evaluating the negative thoughts. Why do these thoughts occur naturally to you? In this stage, one has to question the evidence behind these negative thoughts and also try to identify any unhelpful beliefs that may lead to negative thoughts. Some strategies that one may use in challenging these thoughts are weighing the advantages and disadvantages of worrying or fearing something.

3. Replacing Negative Thoughts with Positive Ones

Once you have challenged these negative thoughts, it is now time to replace these negative thoughts with more realistic and positive thoughts. If this proves hard, one may also find some calming thoughts or words that you can say to yourself if you are facing a situation that causes anxiety.

Managing Stress Self-Help

What is stress?

It refers to a state of emotional or mental strain or tension resulting from adverse or demanding circumstances. While in this state, one feels as if there are very many demanding actions that must be taken while the resources needed are minimal. The strain or tension can be caused by many external factors like illness, work, home, or even family environments. Funnily enough, even those events that are considered joyful, like holidays, can also lead to stress.

Why is managing one's stress helpful? Stress can have a hold on your life, causing you to be sad and thus less productive. It affects your emotional equilibrium and also narrows your ability to think correctly and clearly. Effective stress management can, therefore, go a long way towards relieving a huge burden off your shoulders.

How do you determine whether or not you are under stress? There are various thoughts, emotions, physical sensations, and even behaviors that are associated with this form of mental pressure. Some of these include:

THOUGHTS

- I'll never accomplish this.
- It's not fair. Someone should be helping me.
- This is too much for me.

EMOTIONS

- Angry
- Depressed
- Hopeless
- Impatient

PHYSICAL SENSATIONS

A physical sensation is a physical response to stress and is caused by the body's adrenaline response. Some of the physical feelings associated with stress, therefore are:

- Breathing faster
- Hot and sweaty
- Restless
- Bowel problems, usually short pains

- Difficulty in concentrating because one's mind is focused elsewhere
- A headache

BEHAVIOR

- Lack of sleep
- Lack of appetite
- One is not able to settle
- Use of drugs or even an increase in their use. For example, if one is used to smoking, there will be an increased tendency to smoke

Making Positive Changes

This is aimed at basically managing one's stress levels. Various steps can be followed to make positive changes. They include:

1. Identify the Sources of Stress or the Stressors in Your Life

It's the first step towards making a positive change. This step is not as straightforward as it sounds. Finding the source of chronic stress can be very complicated. To ease things a bit for you, here are some of the questions that you can ask yourself to identify the cause of stress.

- What makes you stressed?
- Where am I when I get stressed?
- What am I doing when I get stressed?
- Who am I with when I get stressed?
- What change can I make?

Some may notice that there is very little that they can do to change some situations. These tiny things could make the difference you need, so do not hesitate to perform them.

2. Identify the Factors that Keep the Problem Going

Once you have identified the sources of your stress, it is now time to identify the factors that keep this problem going.

3. Thinking Differently

This step is fundamentally mental. It means that all you have to change is your thinking towards various situations. To help you improve your thinking, here are some questions that you ought to ask yourself when faced with a particular case:

- What am I reacting to?
- What is it that is going to happen here?
- Is this a fact or an opinion?
- How helpful is it for me to think this way?
- Is it even worth it?
- Am I overestimating the threat?
- What meaning am I giving to this situation?
- What advice would I give to someone else in this situation?
- Can I do things differently here?

Once you have asked yourself these questions and answered them frankly, then you will be able to think positively about a situation.

Doing Things Differently

This step will help with reducing both stress and anxiety. Why? During stress, one usually feels as if many demands cannot be achieved with the available resources. Therefore, doing things differently by maybe considering what applications are most important can help reduce stress levels.

On the other hand, doing things different can help

in reducing anxiety, in that you can now decide to make time for yourself each day to relax or just for fun. One might also choose to create a healthy balance, in that you have time to work, rest, and do other things that concern you.

Tips to Work on Anxiety, Negative Thinking, and Stress

There are several ways of fighting anxiety, negative thinking, and stress:

1. Understand Your Thinking Style

This step right here is the first step to take to change the negative thoughts that one usually has. One must understand how they think precisely. Here are some thinking styles that may help you:

- If you tend to believe that when you fail at one thing, then you have failed at everything, then you are a polarized or black and white thinker.

- If you tend to know what people feel about you and why they act the way they do without them saying so, then you are a person that jumps to conclusions.

- If you tend always to expect disaster to strike no matter what, then you are a catastrophizing thinker. This type of thinker always asks the question: "what if?"

2. The Ability to Recognize Thought Distortions

Once you are able to identify your thinking style, one is able thereby to determine whether it is a thought distortion or not. Types of thought distortions are like those given above in the first step. They include: catastrophizing, making extremely negative predictions, and also making black or white judgments.

3. The Ability to Recognize Rumination

What is rumination? It is a deep or considered thought about something. Typically, when people ruminate, their problem-solving capacity is significantly reduced. Therefore, it is vital for one to recognize this stage during problem-solving and avoid it at all possible costs.

If avoiding ruminating proves to be hard, then the best thing to do when ruminating is to accept that you are having certain thoughts, recognize that they might not be correct, and then allow them to pass in their own mind rather than trying to block them out.

CHAPTER 5
TRIUMPH OVER ANGER AND DEPRESSION

Anger usually occurs as a natural response to feeling attacked, frustrated, or even being humiliated. It is human nature to get angry. The fury, therefore, is not a bad feeling per se, because, at times, it can prove to be very useful. How is this even possible? Anger can open one's mind and help them identify their problems, which could drive one to get motivated to make a change, which could help in molding their lives.

When is Anger a Problem?

Anger, as we have just seen, is normal in life. The problem only comes in when one cannot manage their anger, and it causes harm to people around them or even themselves.

How does one notice when their anger is becoming harmful? When one starts expressing anger through unhelpful or destructive behavior, or even when one's mental and physical health starts deteriorating. That's when one knows that the situation is getting out of hand.

It is the way a person behaves that determines whether or not they have problems with their anger. If the way they act affects their life or relationships, then there is a problem, and they should think about getting some support or treatment.

What is Unhelpful Angry Behavior?

Anger may be familiar to everyone, but people usually express their rage in entirely different ways. How one behaves when they are angry depends on how much control they have over their feelings. People who have less control over their emotions tend to have some unhelpful angry behaviors. These are behaviors that cause damage to themselves or even damage to people or things around them. They include:

Inward Aggression

This is where one directs their anger towards themselves. Some of the behaviors here may include telling oneself that they hate themselves, denying themselves, or even cutting themselves off the world.

Non-Violent or Passive Aggression

In this case, one does not direct their anger anywhere; rather, they stick with the feeling in them. Some of the behaviors here may include ignoring people, refusing to speak to people, refusing to do tasks, or even deliberately doing chores poorly or late. These types of behaviors are usually the worst ways to approach such situations. They may seem less destructive and harmful, but they do not relieve one of the heavy burdens that are causing them to be angry.

Preparation

Weigh Your Options

In life, many things may be out of one's control. These things vary from the weather, the past, other people, intrusive thoughts, physical sensations, and one's own emotions. Despite all these, the power to choose is always disposable to any human. Even though one might not be able to control the weather, one can decide whether or not to wear heavy clothing. One can also choose how to respond to other people.

The first step, therefore, in dealing with anger is to recognize a choice.

Steps to Take in Managing Anger

1. A "Should" Rule is Broken

Everybody has some rules and expectations for one's behavior, and also for other people's behavior. Some of these rules include, "I should be able to do this," "She should not treat me like this," and, "They should stay out of my way." Unfortunately, no one has control over someone else's actions. Therefore, these rules are always bound to be broken, and people may get in one's way. This can result in anger, guilt, and pressure.

It is, therefore, essential to the first break these "should" rules to fight this anger. The first step to make in breaking these rules is to accept the reality of life that someone usually has very little control over other people's lives. The next step is for one to choose a direction based on one's values. How does one know their values? One can identify their values by what angers them, frustrates them, or even enrages them. For example, let's take the rule of "They should stay out of my way." This rule may mean the values of communication, progress, or even cooperation. What do these values mean to someone? Does one have control over them?

Finally, one can act by their values. To help with this, here are two questions one should ask themselves:

- What does one want in the long run?
- What constructive steps can one take in that direction?

2. What Hurts?

The second step is to find the real cause of pain or fear after breaking the rules. These rules usually do not mean the same as one's body. This is because some states of being can hurt one's self-esteem more than others.

To understand this better, let's take the example of Susan, who expects that no one should talk ill of her. Then suddenly John comes up to her and says all manner of things to her. This, therefore, makes Susan enraged. In such a scenario, Susan should ask herself what hurts her. The answer to this question will bring out a general belief about John and herself. She will think that "John is rude," "She is powerless," or even that "She is being made the victim." All these thoughts may hurt her. What may even hurt her most is that she has no control over John's behavior.

Once she has noted that she has no control, she may now consider seeing John's words as a mere opinion rather than an insult. This will make her not see herself as a victim, but as a person just receiving a piece of someone else's mind about herself.

3. Hot Thoughts.

After one has identified what really hurts them, it is now time to identify and, most importantly, replace the hot, anger-driven, and reactive thoughts with more level-headed, more relaxed, and reflective thoughts. Here are some fresh ideas that may be of importance to someone:

Hot thought: "How mean can he be!"

A cool thought: "He thinks he is so caring."

Hot thought: "They are stupid!"

A cool thought: "They are just human."

4. Anger

All the above steps, as one may have noticed, relate to the thoughts. This is because one has first to tackle the ideas before now getting to the emotion. In this step, therefore, one is going to respond to the anger arousal itself. There are three ways that one can follow to respond to this emotion:

- One may indulge in relaxation. This relaxation can come in many forms, like enjoying some music, practicing some progressive muscle relaxation like yoga, and also visualization.

- One may also use that feeling to do some constructive work. When one is angry, there is usually a large amount of energy that one uses at that time. This is the reason that when angry, one can break down things that they would never break when calm. Imagine, therefore, how much that energy would do for someone if just directed to some constructive work.

- One may also try to redefine anger when one gets angry. What does this mean? Once a person is angry, one can try to remind themselves of how anger is a problem that fuels aggression and can cause harm to loved ones and even oneself.

5. Moral Disengagement

In simple words, this step will help one examine the beliefs that turn anger into aggression. These beliefs usually act as mere excuses or justification for destructive acts. Some of these beliefs include "I don't care," "This is the only way I can get my point across," or even "It is high time they recognize me." These beliefs need to be identified early enough and gotten rid of before they can con one into throwing one's morals aside. One sure way of getting rid of them is by reminding oneself of the cost of such beliefs and the advantages of striving for understanding.

6. Aggression

In this step, one now needs to examine the behaviors that arise from aggression and try to fight them. Fighting these behaviors can be achieved if one calms down and puts themselves in the other person's shoes. This will help one understand why the other person is acting in such a manner, what they may be feeling, or even what they may be thinking. This approach will help to:

- Decrease the anger for all parties involved.
- Increase the chance of having a reasonable conversation with the parties involved, and thus everybody is heard.

7. Outcome

The final step of this procedure is to reduce resentment towards others, and also guilt towards oneself.

Treating depression with cognitive behavioral therapy.

What is depression?

Depression is a feeling of severe despondency and dejection. In life, it is only natural for one to feel less than a hundred percent at times. This is like when one is battling with drug addiction or has relationship problems. However, this low feeling sometimes gets a hold of one's life and won't go. This is what we call depression. Depression can make one feel lonely and hopeless.

If one has such feelings, there is light at the end of the tunnel. Cognitive Behavioral Therapy is here to restore one's hope in life. This is because it can help one think more healthily, and also help in overcoming a particular addiction.

Before getting more in-depth with the advantages of CBT on a depressed person, let's first look at the different types of depression.

Types of Depression

Depressions are of various kinds. They can either occur alone or concurrently with an addiction. The best thing, however, is that the following categories are treatable through using CBT.

Major Depression

This disorder occurs when one feels depressed most of the time for most days of the week. Some of the symptoms associated with this disorder are:

- Weight loss or weight gain
- Being tired often
- Trouble getting sleep
- Thoughts of suicide
- Concentration problems
- Feeling restless or agitated

If you experience five or more of the above signs on most days for two weeks or longer, then they have this disorder.

Persistent Depressive Disorder (PDD)

This type of depression usually lasts for two years or even longer. The symptoms associated with the disorder include:

- Sleeping too much or too little
- Fatigue
- Low self-esteem

Bipolar Disorder

A person with such a disorder usually experiences mood episodes that range from extremes of high energy with an "up" mood to low periods.

How CBT Helps with Negative Thoughts of Depression

The cognitive-behavioral therapy understands that when one has low moods, they tend to have negative thinking. This negative thinking usually brings cases of hopelessness, depression, and can also lead to a change in behavior.

CBT, therefore, works to help with the patterns of behavior that need to be changed. In short, it works to recalibrate the part of the brain that keeps a tight hold on happy thoughts.

Five CBT Techniques to Counteract the Negative Thinking of Depression

There are several techniques that one can follow to help with fighting off negative thoughts. Before starting these steps, one should make sure that they are ready to undertake them and should keep track of themselves. Here are some of the steps:

Locate the Problem and Brainstorm for Solutions

The first step is to discover the cause of the problem. This step requires one to talk with one's inner self. Once the idea of what the problem might be dawning on you, write it down in simple words. Then write down a list of things that one can do to improve the problem.

Write Self-Statements to Counteract Negative Thoughts

Once the cause of the problem has been discovered, it is now time to identify the negative thoughts that seem to pop up in one's brain every time. Write self-statements to counteract each foul view. These self-statements are statements that are going to stuff up the negative thoughts. One should always recall all their self-statements and repeat them back to themselves every time a negative thought pops up. However, these self-statements should continually be refreshed because they can, at times, be too routine.

Find New Opportunities to Think Positive Thoughts

Michael is a person who always sees the negative part of people before noticing their bright side. These people, more often than not, usually get depressed quickly. To remedy this, they should always change their thinking and think positively. This, for example, in the case of Michael, can be like first noticing and appreciating how neat people are. This type of thinking can be tough to change. Here are some of the recommended ways that one can adjust to such thinking;

- Set one's phone to remind them to reframe their minds to something positive.

- Pairing up with someone who is working on this same technique. This will make one have positive thoughts, and also get to enjoy them with someone else.

Finish Each Day by Visualizing Its Best Parts

After each day, one can write down the most exciting events of the day and try to remember them. Sharing such moments online can even help one form new associations, and also thinking ways that can prove to be very helpful.

Learn to Accept Disappointment as a Normal Part of Life

In life, disappointment is bound to come one's way. How one deals or behaves after a disappointing event determines how fast one is going to move forward. Take, for example, John, who just lost a job interview. This is a thing that can happen to anyone. The way he responds to this situation will determine how fast he is going to move forward. If he starts getting the thoughts of "I am a failure," "The world is so unfair to me," or even "I will never succeed in life," then he is moving in the wrong direction. Later, he can write some things he has learned from the experience and things he can do to remedy it next time.

CHAPTER 6
ESSENTIAL COGNITIVE BEHAVIOR THERAPY TECHNIQUES

Socratic Questioning

This method involves asking more than telling the patient. This is an extremely tool that allows the patient to go through all the possible negative feelings and thoughts they may have, end come to the surface. It is encouraged to let them express what they feel inside until they are ready to change their own minds. The professional is just there to guide the patient to the realization that they had been wrong all along. His or her work is not to provide a therapeutic reframe where they provide solutions; they think it is best for the client. These solutions may be driven by emotions and may be full of personal or emotional bias. People are more likely to rebel against things that they deem untrue and an inaccurate representation of their situation.

There are, however, more likely to accept their own representation of conclusions they draw for themselves. He or she may ask if their way of thinking applies to all situations in her life and allow them to expound on their answer. He or she can include possibilities in the way they frame the question like is it possible that you are making an assumption about your situation? It allows the practitioner to introduce their own way of thinking in a way that the patient can be receptive as it forces them to think before giving an answer. He or she allows the patient to give more reasons that they think the way they do. All this is done by strategic questioning that helps the patient define their core values as he or she explains to the practitioner who they are as a person.

Journaling

There is power in putting down your thoughts down on paper when you start to feel that they are affecting you. It is like a mind dump where you empty what you are feeling, and then you start feeling lighter. It could be used to record habits, moods, thoughts, emotions, and their intensity. It can also include how we responded when we were faced with certain situations. By having a visual representation of our thoughts, we can be able to recognize them and find ways in which we can change or cope with them.

Homework

This technique is frequently applied to cognitive restructuring, where the patient gets some tasks they can do at home, similar to school homework. They take their assignment home and work on what had been learned from the practitioner. Examples of homework a person may receive may include behavior activation or tracking their automatic thoughts for a day. Whatever the tasks assigned, they should be done until the next time the patient and practitioner meet. During the session, they will both participate in analyzing what the patient put down and discuss more about it. More often than not, the patient will have realized something by putting it down that will trigger their mind toward sharing and eventually healing.

Relaxed Breathing

Relaxed breathing is mainly taught through meditation that shall be discussed later in the book. When one is taught relaxed breathing, they are also taught to clear out the baggage they have in their minds and keep focusing on something as simple as breathing. It helps with anxiety as one is able to clear out negative thinking and appreciate relaxing by breathing in and out repeatedly.

Using Reflective Reframing

Here, the aim is not to give advice or opinions to the patient, but rather, it is to encourage them to keep sharing by asking questions. One, it is important for clarification in case we have not understood what the patient is talking about. Two, it is the basis of trust when the patient notices you are listening to them and engaging them in conversation. Therapy is not just about listening and letting the other person spill their guts, it's like a conversation between friends where there is no judgment but support no matter what.

Successful Approximation

This is the perfect technique for procrastinators and people that find it difficult to complete a task once they have started it. This can be because they don't have the necessary skills to complete the tasks, they may also feel overwhelmed and decide not to complete the task, or they are just people who start and never complete anything. This technique encourages the patient to look at the task as smaller, simpler tasks that can be accomplished with ease. Once he or she masters those, they won't see the bigger task as something to be scared of.

Unraveling Cognitive Distortions

Decentering

This technique works best for people that care so much what other people think, especially in the negative. It allows the person to explain why they think this is always the case with them and then focuses on remoting this king of thought by encouraging them to do the things they are putting off out of fear and see if people actually think negatively about them. It can also involve encouraging the patient to ask a question instead of assuming what other people are thinking. They can be taught how to communicate better to get to the root of the problem.

Behavior Experiments

This technique involves challenging the way one behaves on a day to day basis. It involves looking at how the patient observes things, how he reflects upon situations, the way they plan for the future, and what they are experiencing. The way this is done is through a series of tests and discovery, a set of activities that help these behaviors come to light or simply just observing how the patient reacts and responds during a session. The therapist gets a feel of the person and jots down what they think and the best possible way they can help the patient recovery. What works for one patient may not for the next. It is up to the patient to discern and tailor-make a treatment that will benefit the patient fully.

When a practitioner discovers a negative thought that recurs—for example, a person sees themselves as a failure—they will try to get to the root of the problem through a series of experiments which could benefit the patient by allowing them to see that this shouldn't be a general way of thinking. It allows them to see that by thinking like this, they will still face failure in the future, but this kind of blanket thinking is unnecessary and even false. Here, the practitioner can introduce positive affirmations to counter the negative thoughts that the patient may have.

Systemic Desensitization

When a practitioner learns more about a person, they can also learn their triggers and why they feel the way they do. In having this information, he or she can have some sessions where the patient is made for relaxing, and a triggering stimulus is introduced. The patient will react the way they normally do, but the practitioner will talk them through the anxiety they are feeling to a point they are able to relax again. Through constant exposure, the triggers will slowly lose their grip on the mental state of the patient and eventually disappear with a lot more work.

Thought Records/Self-Monitoring

Here, a patient keeps a detailed record of the way they feel, their habits, the way they think over some time. It is almost similar to homework, but the patient is doing most of the work. It could be an extension of homework where the patient feels like they still require to keep a record of the negative thoughts or emotions that they are constantly feeling. It is like keeping a diary, and the therapist can be involved in helping the patient analyze the different issues that arise.

Treating Thoughts as Guesses

This technique is very useful, especially for people that are affected by negative thoughts. Negative thoughts have a way of creeping in and making every problem appear bigger than it is. It makes people seem like they are the problem or our own selves as the problem. This technique allows us to demystify that every thought that goes through our minds as facts but to treat them as guesses. This allows us not to jump into conclusion or put our formed bias in the final decision we make. For example, if the mind says that we should be getting a promotion because we have worked so hard the past couple of years, we should take that as a guess because we don't know what evaluations were made when choosing the person who got promoted. This makes us accept things that are out of our control and make us more active in finding out facts before jumping into conclusions. It encourages us to use the logical part of our brains as opposed to simple thoughts that summarize a complex problem in a short sentence.

Scheduling Pleasant Activities/Activity Scheduling

For a person that is always thinking that everything is bad and nothing good ever happens, they would benefit from putting down the days of the week and planning at least one peasant activity that they enjoy and do it every day. This may be quite difficult for a person that is severely depressed; therefore, they can start with the most basic things, such as going outside in the sun, and they can graduate to more complex stuff depending on how well they are progressing. Another way to approach this is by putting down activities that give a sense of gratification or mastery afterward. It can be taking cooking lessons or learning a new language; whatever it is, one should start with a few minutes and keep increasing the time as they develop a habit.

This technique gives someone something to live for every day. With time it shall become like a part of who they are. It also allows one to focus on the good emotions lie joy, anticipation, happiness, hope that comes with having something pleasant to do every day. With time patients and be able to schedule more than one activity per day. They should, however, be advised against multitasking. Each activity should be done on its own, and I should be emphasized that it's okay not to feel like doing them once in a while. Acknowledging that will lead to a kinder way of dealing with disappointment in oneself.

Progress Muscle Relaxation (PMR)

This technique involves staying still and listening to your body. Release all tension you may be experiencing and bring your body to a state of total relaxation. Let your muscles relax by using professional guidance, relaxation tapes, videos, or your mind. This practice is very common in mindfulness, where the patient gets to let go of everything that is burdening them and lets their body experience perfect serenity. It is not an easy practice as it can take a long time before someone is able to let go and just be relaxed. The results left one sharp and focused and without the burden of negative thoughts.

Cognitive Restructuring

This technique makes people confront their negative thought patterns and how they affect their way of thinking or are responsible for their bad habits. It deals with the core beliefs that a person has learned over time and tries to change those negative thoughts into positive thoughts. A person has first to acknowledge that these negative thoughts exist and spend some time putting them down in a thought record form. They can then realize a pattern and look for a more positive approach, such as positive affirmations. It involves changing a person from the inside, which will then reflect on the outside.

Skills Training

Skill training embraces the learning aspect of things. It encourages the patient to learn and get the skills they require so that they can do what they want. For example, if a person wants to become a car salesman, developing skills like communication and negotiation can be vital to realize their goals eventually. Learning new skills gives a person a sense of accomplishment. The practitioner teaches these skills by role-playing activities and modeling or teaches them directly to the patient.

Exposure Therapy

This CBT technique encourages approaching problems rather than avoiding them. The reason people develop anxiety and depression is that they are afraid of confronting what they are most afraid of. Through a series of guided exposure experiments, patients are encouraged to confront their fear and let it go, starting from the most basic to the more challenging ones. Exposure therapy encourages on to be in the presence of things or situation that causes fear for them for some time until when its effects reduce. Regular practice is recommended for maximum results.

I. Interoceptive Exposure

This technique involving the patient's body sensations that cause fear and anxiety for some time. He or she will respond to the sensation, but the exposure is maintained without interruptions. The person is encouraged to notice what they think when they are exposed to this sensation and to gain a new understanding of it. The patient then realizes that there is nothing to fear, and the anxiety is unfounded.

II. Nightmare Exposure and Rescripting

This is similar to interoceptive exposure but with nightmares.

III. Situation Exposure Therapy

The patient is encouraged to write down situations they would normally avoid on paper and write down the level of anxiety you feel when you think about each one of those scenarios. Arrange these situations in descending order and have the patient confront the theme of the list they have created. This should be an indicator of the problems they have.

IV. Imagery based Exposure

Here, the patient is asked to recall a recent memory in which they felt the strongest emotion. He or she is then asked to describe what they remember in detail, be it the environment, what they experienced in terms of senses, etc. They are then asked to pinpoint what they felt using a verb and what they wanted to do at that moment. The practice is repeated until they feel less distressed than they originally were.

Mindfulness Practice

We shall discuss mindfulness practices in full later in the book, but in summary, mindfulness allows the patient to allow in everything that they are feeling and let it pass through them. They can then acknowledge what they feel and accept it.

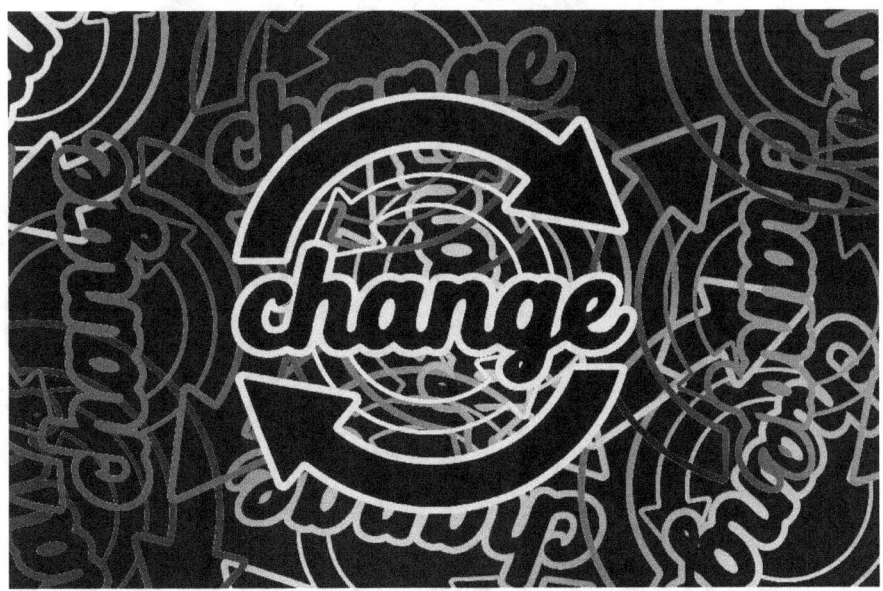

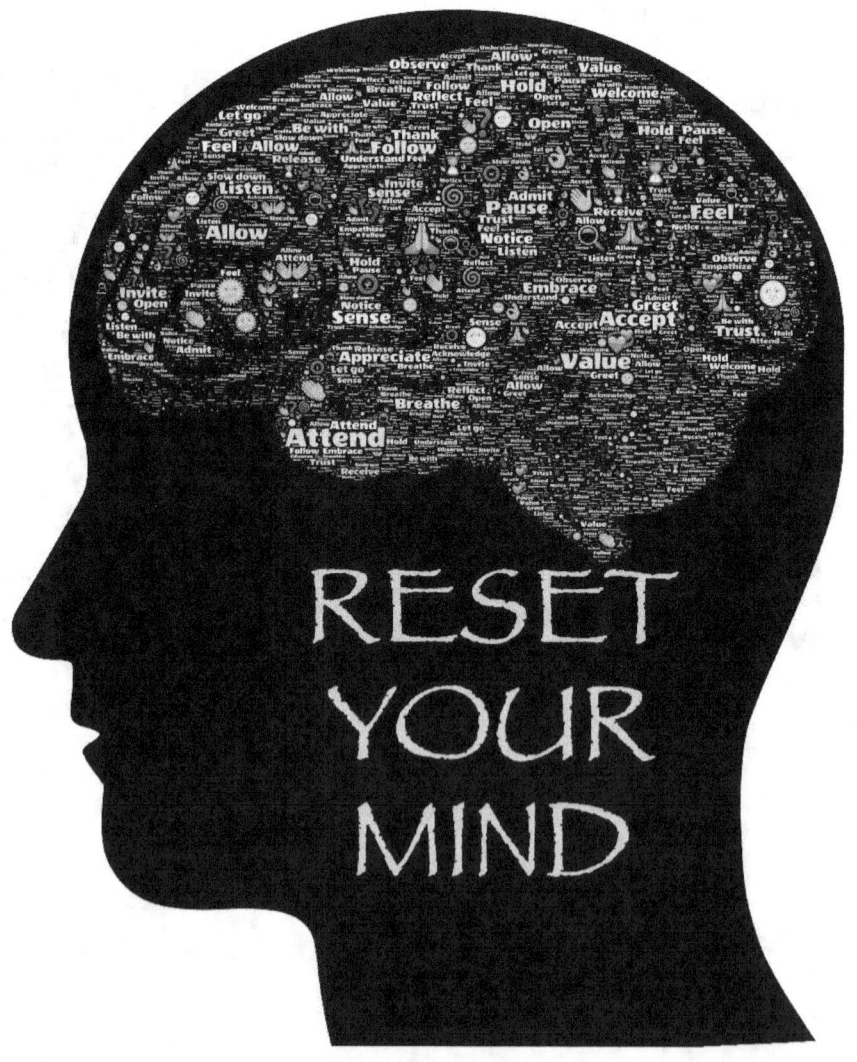

CHAPTER 7
COGNITIVE BEHAVIORAL TREATMENTS FOR ANXIETY

In this chapter, you will learn about two methods that have been shown to have the best results for anxiety disorders.

Relaxation Training

You can also adapt those strategies to treat anxiety as well. Here are some additional relaxation techniques you can use:

- **Yoga or Stretching:** an exercise form like yoga or stretching, which forces you to slow down and become aware of the sensations in your body, is a great way to manage your anxiety. There are a number of reasons for this. First of all, it's slow-paced, but it can also be rigorous so that your overactive and anxious mind is still occupied with the activity rather than straying to other topics.

Secondly, it both slows and strengthens your heart while opening up your veins to improve circulation. All of this contributes to a decrease in the physical symptoms of anxiety, which will make it much easier to manage the mental and emotional symptoms.

- **Meditation:** meditation is a great way to improve self-awareness and concentration while decreasing stress. It will help strengthen your mind so that you are better armed against stressful situations. You can find many free guides to meditation online or buy a book, video, or another training course to help you learn how to do it.

Acceptance and Commitment Therapy

There are four major stages to Acceptance and Commitment Therapy (ACT) that make it well suited for helping you manage anxiety (as well as depression and even addiction).

- **Awareness:** the first step (which you might have noticed is similar to many first steps in the previous methods) is to improve self-awareness. Pay attention to the links between thoughts, emotions, and behaviors. What thoughts contribute to your anxiety? What behaviors relate to your anxiety? How do these thoughts and behaviors make you feel?

- **Acceptance:** the next (and one of the hardest) steps is acceptance. Rather than blame yourself or feel ashamed that you have a problem with anxiety, learn to accept it. This doesn't mean you continue to be anxious. Rather, accept that you are not perfect (and that *nobody* is). Accept the whole of your being (this includes your strengths as well, not just your weaknesses).

- **Goal Setting:** determine reasonable goals that you are passionate about. If you want to get further in your career, for example, figure out exactly how your anxiety is preventing you from doing that and come up with an actionable plan for overcoming your anxiety so that you can achieve your goals.

- **Committed Action:** in summary, this step asks you to just get to it! Once you have become more self-aware and created a realistic plan for achieving your goals, the only thing left to do is get out there and start doing! Commit yourself to act on your goals. Create daily tasks that you can manage to complete that will bring you closer to where you want to be and who you want to be.

CHAPTER 8
COGNITIVE BEHAVIORAL TREATMENTS FOR DEPRESSION

Of all the disorders that currently exist, depression has, by far, seen the most successful results from cognitive behavioral therapy. This form of treatment has actually proven to be as effective as taking antidepressant medication.

In this chapter, you will learn two strategies that have proven to be the most effective in the treatment of depression:

Cognitive Processing Therapy

    1. Identify past traumatic experience(s): one major fact of depression is usually some form of traumatic experience in the past (whether it is abuse, a divorce, or another upsetting event). If you did not allow yourself (or otherwise did not have the opportunity) to process the pain and emotions at the time, then those are likely still plaguing you to this day. The first step could take a while for some people. And everyone is going to feel uncomfortable or afraid to dig these things back up. But you must act like the reckless explorer in uncharted waters, boldly following the current, wherever it takes you. Go deep into yourself and really see what is there. You can do this in the privacy of your own mind, so you don't have to worry about others learning what is there without your permission.

2. **Become aware of thoughts and feelings:** once you have identified your traumatic experience(s). You need to explore them even further. What feelings come up to the surface as you think about them? There are two exercises you need to do for this step.

First, you need to write a detailed description of the experiences. Write every single thing you can remember. You don't have to show it to anyone. Just write it down. This act of writing it helps extract it from you as if you were surgically slicing it out of yourself. You take power from it. But it does not get the whole job done. The second exercise is to read that description again, add more details if you remember more. Then, on a new sheet of paper, write down what emotions come up for you now. What was the experience of reading it like for you on an emotional level?

3. **Learn new coping skills:** at this point, you are pretty raw and probably feeling as if you had been freshly cut open. This step should last the longest as retraining yourself to use new coping skills is a rigorous process that takes commitment and dedication.

4. **Understand the changes in yourself:** when the new coping skills start to feel a little more like a habit, take some time to do a follow-up assessment. Read the description of the traumatic experience again. What feelings come up for you now? How is your emotional experience now different than it was before?

Cognitive Therapy

1. **Track your negative thoughts:** use the example at the end of this chapter to make your own thought record for your negative thoughts whenever you have a negative thought, briefly note it in your record. Try to

make this a daily habit. Keep the record on your phone or in a notebook that you can carry with you so that it is easy to access.

2. **Become aware of cognitive distortions:** at the end of each day, note what sort of cognitive distortion(s) can be associated with each negative thought you had throughout the day. Note this down next to the thought. Doing this regularly it will help you to become more aware of your thoughts and what's really behind them.

3. **Look for positives:** after about 1 or 2 weeks of just repeating the first two steps on a daily basis, add this third step to your routine. After you have finished with your daily analysis of cognitive distortions, write down at least one positive thing about your day. It doesn't matter how small it might seem. The purpose of this exercise is to train your brain to start finding the positives in your day. They *are* there. Gradually increase the challenge by trying to add more and more positive things each day.

CHAPTER 9
COGNITIVE DISTORTION

One of the most recognizable causes of depression is the distortions of the mind. A way of thinking that our minds have need accustomed to either from birth or learned through society as we grow up. Cognitive distortions are a topic that came to light through the research of two brilliant psychiatrists called Aaron Beck and David Burns. Depression is, in most cases, a series of negative thoughts that gnaw away at one's self-worth and self-esteem for a long period. Cognitive distortions or styles of negative thinking, by definition, are negative thinking habits that are often untrue or exaggerated that cause a person to misrepresent events. The reason these irrational thoughts are so dangerous is that they are seldom recognizable until later in one's life when it's really hard to change them. Notice that I have said difficult, not impossible.

These are the characteristics of cognitive distortions:

They are a habitual way of thought and belief.

They are always untrue.

They are likely to cause a psychological problem like stress, anxiety, or depression in the future.

We have already discussed that cognitive behavior therapy can be a solution for cognitive distortions. In this chapter, we are going to have an in-depth discussion about cognitive distortions and how to deal with them.

Black-and-White Thinking/Polarized Thinking/All-or-Nothing Thinking

Here, a person only perceives things in two extremes, either good or bad. In his or her mind, there cannot be another way of looking at things. They dwell more on these extremes, even if there is another angle to view the problem. This kind of thinking doesn't just affect the person with distorted thoughts; it affects the people around them too. The person will always look at people's views as wrong or right. This makes it hard for them to agree with other people during discussions as they cannot see the grey area is issues. I know an ethical problem with thoughts called the Trolley Problem. In this case, there is a runaway trolley heading to a junction in which one side has five people tied on the train tracks, and on the other side, there is just one person tied to the train tracks. The question is which of these choices would be the right one? The black and white thinker would pick one of the two, the problem goes ahead to introduce more scenarios that would make a choice "easier by the wrong" nonetheless. The problem with this type of thinking is that situations or people cannot be boxed by simple solutions. One has to critically think before making assumptions or decisions regarding problems presented before them. The same applies to oneself; you are not a success if you are rich or a failure if you are poor. You are much more than these two adjectives.

Solution:

This person needs to understand that there are no situations that can have two extreme solutions. First, they should start by eliminating "never "and "always" from how they speak or think about scenarios.

Then, they should consider a proper representation of the scenario and adopt it in their thinking and speaking.

Mental Filtering

A person may have a hundred things going right for him or her in this situation. Instead, they will choose to focus on that one thing that had gone wrong. To them, the negative takes center stage regardless of any positives that may have come before it. For example, a bride may have had a beautiful wedding by all standards, but the decorator used the wrong shade of the theme color she had chosen. If she has mental filtering, despite the successful and beautiful wedding, she will choose to sulk and complain about that small detail that too many others didn't affect any part of the day negatively. In short, a person cannot appreciate the good things if they are not perfect.

Solution:

Everyone has to pinpoint what really matters in their life. Mental filters hinder you from enjoying the positive and affect those around you as you will transfer your negative energy to them. Always choose to look at the bright side of things.

Overgeneralization

In this situation, a person has a general rule for certain people for the situation. The rule may have applied once or twice before in the person's life, and after that, they have made it an assumption that it is true for that situation. They frequently use the words "always" and "never" when talking. For example, a student that studies hard may fail two consecutive final exams. Instead of thinking maybe the papers were set in areas he or she had not studied or look at the general performance of other students, his or her mind does to "I will never pass this subject." Overgeneralization prevents a person from looking at other reasons that something happened because they have already predetermined the results. They will, therefore, quit or putting effort because their way of thinking says no matter the effort, nothing can change. I can associate this kind of thinking with the character Eeyore from *Winnie the Pooh*, the children's cartoon.

Solution:

Acknowledge people's personalities and individuality. The same also applies to situations and events. Be adaptable when the situation changes and have an open mind when it comes to making decisions.

Jumping to Conclusions

This kind of thinking involves making assumptions prematurely before all the facts are revealed. A person thinks of the worst before things become clear to them. In most cases, this type of thinking comes when a person has experienced disappointment before. They may have some deep-seated trust issues that one has not dealt with.

A good example of this is a person that is constantly suspicious that their partner is cheating when they choose to talk privately on the phone or have a protective password on their applications. The partner may not have wanted to distract the other person and thought it was polite to pick the call outside. He or she may have a password protected phone for security and may share with their partner if only they asked. Jumping to a conclusion is bad because people make rash decisions out of emotions (e.g., some people stab a partner they suspect of cheating in a fit of rage).

Solutions:

Choose to always listen to explanations before making a decision. If you are prone to anger, withdraw from the situation, and revisit it once you are calm and can be able to think properly. There is no harm in giving people the benefit of the doubt, but don't allow yourself to be lied to or make excuses when you know your instincts are right.

Labelling and Mislabeling

Here, you may use the wrong labels to represent who you are because of a scenario. The labeling and mislabeling don't accurately represent who you are just because something has gone wrong. An example is when a person starts a business, and it fails within the first year. Inappropriate labeling would be he or she is a bad businessman/businesswoman. They forget that there are so many factors that could have led to the collapse of the business that had nothing to do with them as a person. Maybe the timing wasn't right to start the business. Maybe customers didn't need the product at that time. Maybe there was a recession. Maybe they had not researched on who their target audience was. There are so many maybes that have nothing to do with the person at all.

Solution:

Know how to detach your personality from a setback. Take negatives as a lesson that shows you what not to do next time. Pick labels that represent who you want to be.

Personalization

Personalization comes when someone associates someone else's actions with who they are. They take on the responsibility of another person to be as a reflection of their efforts or lack thereof. This type of thinking happens to parents and children. A parent may take a child's failure or injury as a reflection of who they are as a parent. A child may fail to achieve what their parent wants and blame themselves. When a person is emotionally attached to another person, they are more likely to take the other person's failures as their own, which is wrong.

Solution:

It is vital to remember that everyone, as an individual, should take responsibility for their own life. If a student fails in school, it doesn't represent how they were raised; instead, it shows that they didn't work hard. A child who does things just to please his or her parents will fail because that's not who they are.

Emotional Reasoning

Sometimes thinking with our emotions rather than logically can bring negative effects onto our lives. This is when someone puts so much weight on their emotions when they are making important decisions. One may make a decision not to do something just because they don't feel like doing it. This is called procrastination. Another person may go out with a person they don't like because they feel sorry for them. Another person may fail to pursue their dreams because of what other people may think about them. Emotional reasoning prevents a person from moving forward.

Solution:

Thinks logically instead of emotionally. Sometimes fears may just be in your head, and when you make a logical decision, you will find out that what you feared was just a mirage.

Should statements

This type of thinking places the importance of our way of thinking instead of considering other people. We think things should be done a certain way regardless. We fail to recognize that what works for us doesn't necessarily work for everyone else. Consider a statement, "She is so beautiful. She should be married by now." This is wrong because we are not them and don't know the struggle this individual is battling, hence her singleness. She may be working on herself before getting married.

Solution:

Stop passing your judgment on other people instead of work on your own reality. After all, there is nothing you can do about what another person's choices or issues.

Double Standard

Some people have a false sense of self-importance. They don't think that what applies to other people should apply to them and vice versa. This is where people who think they are better than other people because they are from a certain economic background, gender race, religion, country, and so on.

It includes the false belief that some things apply to you and later changes when it no longer suits you. For example, one may say the support that everyone should be taxed according to their income, but when you realize that you may be taxed more because you have a larger income, you change your mind. This type of thinking makes some people choose what suits them even if it affects other people.

Solution:

Think of everyone as equal and deserves the same treatment. Putting yourself in another person's shoes can be an effective way to understand people's struggles and change your attitude toward people that are different.

Blaming Others/Denying Responsibility

This has become rampant in today's society when everyone feels it's everyone else's fault rather than acknowledge they are part of the problem. Some people make choices, and when things go wrong, they choose to point an accusing finger at the other person rather than accept responsibility. Think of a person that is an alcoholic and chooses to blame the brewing company for advertising their product. Sometimes blaming others can affect the people around you because it takes too much time that could be spent finding a solution. This is common when leaders make a mistake and pride get in the way.

Solution:

Taking responsibility can be hard, but you will find people respecting you more for it. Spend less time making excuses and more time looking for appropriate actions you can take to make the situation better.

Magical Thinking

Here, a person assumes that things would be better if only this or that happened. A person thinks that the grass is greener on the other side. An example is when a person looks at magazines and thinks that they would be happy if they were rich, skinny, or beautiful. These slowly fuels self-esteem and negative self-image. It can lead someone to take extreme measures such as cosmetic surgeries to enhance their physical appearance, eating disorders to become skinny, or dating older men or women with money to get rich. Magical thinking fuels one thinks that good things can be acquired in a short amount of time with little effort.

Solution:

Think of yourself as an individual whose time is yet to come. Look for triggers that make you have this type of thinking and keep away from them. Do a social media cleanse if you are constantly comparing yourself to others and work on yourself. Set goals and work toward achieving them without looking for shortcuts.

Fallacies

Fallacies are the wrong way in which we perceive things. Some fallacies are engrained in us associated with negative thinking. One is the fallacy of change when one assumes, and they would be better off if another person changes their behavior. This is a selfish way of thinking and leads to disappointment because many people will not change who they are to accommodate us. The second one is a fallacy of fairness when one assumes that they deserve fairness and equality when sometimes it's not the case. The third one controls fallacy when a person insists on constantly being in control over everything.

Solution:

One has to acknowledge that they can only change things about themselves and not what other people do. The element of control of situations, events, or people is impossible, and they may not work how one wants them to. Acceptance of these facts reduces the pressure that one has on others to perform.

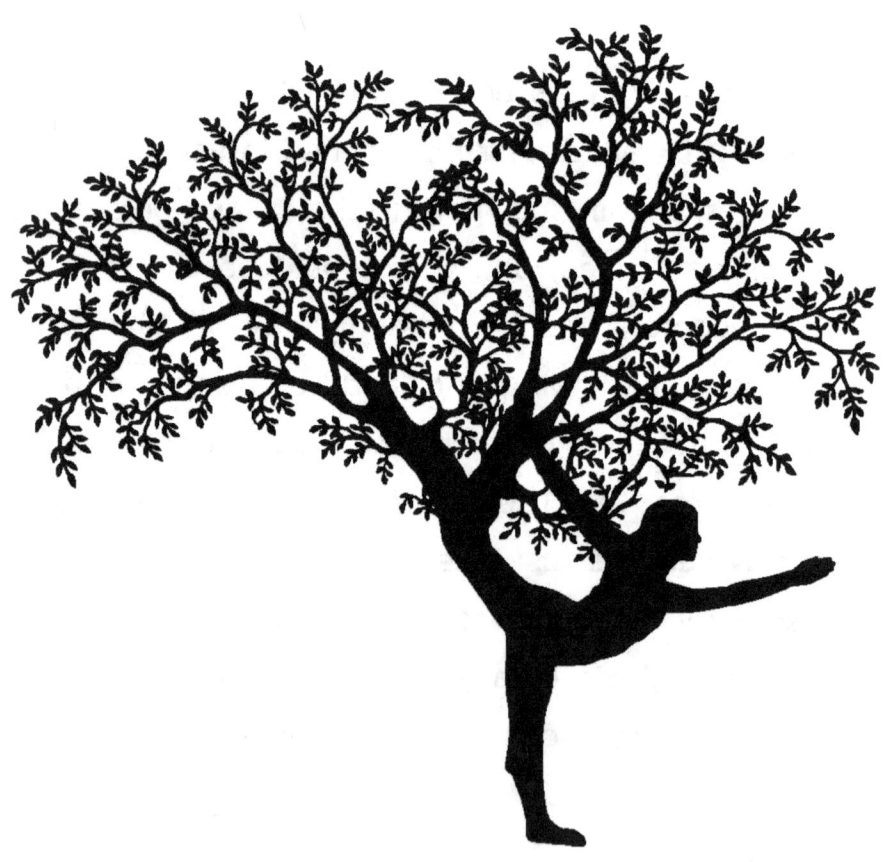

CHAPTER 10
USE THE RIGHT KIND OF EXERCISE

We all know that exercise is very beneficial for the human species. A ton of studies and experts have pointed that out to us. However, some "experts" have been preaching some unhealthy principles of exercise, which has unfortunately caused billions of people to look at exercise in a way that doesn't necessarily benefit their bodies, health, and certainly not stress levels.

Recommending certain types of exercises can be very controversial because there are many different opinions out there, and many of them are based on pseudoscience or studies that don't even exist. In this book, we will use a science-based approach that allows you to do enjoyable and relaxing exercises, which will both benefit your stress levels and optimize your health.

Exercise and chronic stress have a weird relationship. On the one hand, we all know that regular exercise has a large number of health benefits. However, on the other hand, you will know that exercising too much can also cause chronic stress.

Too much or too little?

I believe there are just as many people in the Western world who exercise too much as there are people who exercise too little. Furthermore, exercising too much is just as bad for your health, if not worse, than exercising too little. When you exercise too much, your body raises cortisol. This is called overtraining and is a form of chronic stress. As you know, when cortisol rises, your stress response is on, which will naturally make you feel stressed and tired.

Overtraining has many of the same side effects as chronic stress because the physical reaction is pretty much the same. Overtraining will leave you extremely fatigued and oftentimes even depressed. Exercising too much is one of the last things you want to do if you suffer from chronic stress. However, not exercising at all is also very unhealthy, so you should not avoid exercise entirely either.

Instead, you want to find that "sweet spot" where you get the amazing health benefits of regular exercise while you avoid exercising too much and the unwanted side effects that come with that. The keys to finding this sweet spot are to listen to your body and create a balanced exercise program that leaves you feeling energized, not tired, after performing it.

If you have a wearable device that can measure your heart rate and/or heart rate variability, these can also be great to use to check if you have been exercising too much and if you have recovered properly, so that you're ready to exercise more. If your heart rate drops quickly during the night and if your HRV is high during the night, these are signs that you are recovering well. If your heart rate lowers late and your HRV is low during the night, you should probably not go for a physically challenging exercise program the next day. Instead, you should simply relax and recover. However, in this book, we are going to assume that you just listen to your body. That's the free solution, and it often works just fine for our purpose of relieving stress.

So, how can you listen to your body? It's pretty simple. There are two rules that you should follow if you want your exercise routine to lower stress rather than raise it.

The first rule is: If you feel too fatigued to exercise, don't do it. Spending hours on a treadmill will just make you more fatigued. If you do want to get some exercise in that situation, it should be low-level physical activity, which doesn't put too much stress on your body.

The second rule is: If you feel like you have less energy after exercising than you had before, you have been exercising too hard or too much. When lower stress is your goal, exercising should always give you more energy, not less.

These are the two exercise rules to keep in mind when you exercise to lower stress levels. When you are chronically stressed, you don't want to do anything that puts more stress on your body, which is exactly what exercising too hard or for too long does. Instead, you want to do something that is enjoyable and makes you feel good afterward. Now that you know what the main principles of your stress-relieving exercise routine should be let's take a look at which types of exercise you can use to get the best benefits for your stress levels and your health.

Low-level Physical Exercise

low-level physical activity can offer some great benefits, and I recommend that you use this type of exercise as much as you like, as long as your body is okay with it. These types of exercises are least likely to worsen stress. Rather, they should feel very relaxing.

Low-level physical exercise can be a walk, a yoga session, an easy bike ride, a hike, or anything else that isn't very physically challenging. Doing low-level physical exercise every day can be very good for your stress levels, and it doesn't have to be that difficult. All you have to do is walk around for a bit (preferably in nature).

Resistance Training

If you have the energy for it, doing some resistance training once in a while can be very good for your resilience to stress and your overall health.

Resistance training is when your body pushes against a force. The most common types of resistance training are weight lifting and other types of strength training. It sounds stressful for the body to do some heavy weight lifting, you might think. And you would be completely right. However, it is a bit more complex than that.

Resistance training does put some stress on your

body in the short term. This is not necessarily a bad thing if you have a proper routine, though. The key to a proper resistance training routine is enough recovery time. I recommend six to nine days. When you do resistance training this way, you will make your body momentarily stressed after the exercise. However, when you allow your body to recover for six to nine days, it will increase your resilience to stress in the long term. So, when you follow this routine, you exchange some short-term stress for long-term stress relief and resistance.

However, if you're already very stressed, you might not want the momentary stress increase from resistance training. That's why I recommend that you only do resistance training if you feel like you have enough energy to do it. If you do, it can be very beneficial for you and make you more resilient to stress over time.

Aerobic Exercise

Aerobic exercise is very popular, and it can be beneficial. However, it can also require a lot of effort and time, which can be quite stressful.

Aerobic exercise, also known as endurance training or cardio, can be something like running, swimming, or cycling. Or it can be almost any sports that require constant movement. If you have an existing practice of this type of exercise that you like, you can keep doing that. Especially if it also includes good social relationships. However, aerobic exercise is typically not the first type of exercise that I would recommend for people with chronic stress issues. That's because endurance training is oftentimes seen as something you must do every day, or at least three to four times a week, for 30-60 minutes to get good results. This can be a lot of time for you to invest, which you really don't have to. Plus, it can be very taxing for your body and just put more stress on it. Also, you really don't have to do aerobic exercise for several hours every week to see good benefits from your exercise routine.

Like I said, if you have an aerobic exercise that you like that makes you feel better, you can keep doing that. However, I would only do aerobic exercise several times a week for the fun it could provide, not necessarily for the benefits. If you have fun doing it, it can be great. However, if you just want the health benefits and better resilience to stress in a short time as possible, there are better ways.

HIIT

High-intensity interval training (HIIT) gives you a combination of the good effects of aerobic exercise and resistance training in a very short amount of time. It improves your mitochondria; it helps with detoxification and weight loss and dramatically increases growth hormone levels. In other words, it is perhaps the best way to exercise for your health.

In a HIIT workout, you shift between doing high-intensity intervals and resting. For example, you can sprint for 60 seconds and then sit or lie down for 90 seconds. And when I say sprint, I really mean sprint. You want to get some real effort into those 60 seconds, so your heart rate rises as much as possible. Because when your heart rate is high, you will get the benefits of aerobic exercise while you're relaxing between the intervals.

However, HIIT doesn't have to be running. It can be anything that allows you to do a high-intensity interval and get your heart rate up quickly. The best thing about HIIT is that it takes very little time. You simply do the intervals for as long as you can, or for a maximum of 15 minutes in total. This means that you will, at most, be doing six sprints or other high-intense intervals. Furthermore, you only have to do this once a week. Just once a week will give you amazing benefits. You don't have to put more time into it. When you combine HIIT with low-level physical activity throughout the week, your exercise routine will require almost no time, and it will give a whole bunch of benefits. Your resilience to stress should also increase significantly.

Again, it's important to mention that you should always listen to your body. If your fatigue becomes worse after doing HIIT, it might not be the right thing for you at that moment. If that is the case, you can try to do HIIT later when you are less stressed. However, as with resistance training, HIIT should only put stress on your body in the short term, whereas it should increase your resilience to stress in the long term.

Generally, HIIT is very beneficial, and it probably won't hurt you to try it once. You can just do one high-intensity interval for 60 seconds and see how you feel the next day or a few days after. If you feel better, you can go for more the following week. If you feel worse, you might want to wait some extra time before you try it again. Recover

When it comes to exercising, the most important thing you can do to minimize stress is to ensure that your body is fully recovered after a workout before you start a new one. If you feel like your body isn't fully recovered after exercising, you should relax or only do some light movement until you're fully recovered.

CHAPTER 11
YOU ARE YOUR OWN CURE

Living with anxiety means that you are always on edge. You're living a life that is propelled by fear. This makes it difficult to find any type of enjoyment to speak of. Your mind is always stuck on the "what ifs" that may happen. Rather than being able to live in the moment, all your thoughts are directed either on the guilt of the past or the unpredictable prospects of the future.

This is no way to live, and the fact that you're reading this book shows that you don't want to continue to live that way. An anxiety disorder is a common occurrence in today's modern world. Things move fast, and the ability to take your time and relish at the moment is fleeting at best. However, it is comforting to know that you don't have to live that way. You can do something about it.

Google anxiety, and you will be immediately inundated with options of all kinds. Some will promise to heal you through herbs and diets, others offer you a wide array of medications, and then some will tell you just to slough it off, and things will get better. You and I both know and understand that your choices for reclaiming your life are many.

While there has been a great deal of success in many of these methods, we encourage you to attempt to resolve your anxiety issues in a more natural way. Your brain and your body have already been designed to heal itself. It's just that most of us have lost touch with how to communicate with our bodies effectively. We go through life like an automaton, jumping from one function to another, void of feelings and confidence. However, if we learn to tap into our own natural resources, health and recovery are often just a short distance away.

The reality is that we have the power to heal ourselves within us. In most cases, you won't need expensive medications, pay hundreds of dollars to therapists, or buy into a lot of expensive gadgetry. There are steps you can take right now, techniques you can apply the moment you feel your anxiety start to rise to help your mind to reach a calmer state so you can add more positive feelings to your life.

Getting in the Right Frame of Mind

Regardless of the method, you choose to aid you in recovery, keep these basic points in mind before you begin any treatment. We live in a world full of negativity, so it's no wonder that we drift off into the negativity of land without effort. The challenge, though, is to redirect our thoughts to the more positive. This will be the first step in getting our thinking back on track.

Show Gratitude: Cultivate a spirit of gratitude.

Believe it or not, this is a mental exercise that all of us can practice. This is not just to be thankful for the basic things in life but to think deeper in that same line of thought. Making a concerted effort to at least feel gratitude inside can start us thinking more positively.

Our world is rushed, and often, we don't take the time to appreciate the things we receive without asking. Good health, a family that cares, a regular paycheck, or just being able to have a meal on the table. In the beginning, you may have to set up reminders to stop and show your appreciation for what you have.

We are all accustomed to using cues to remind us of other activities, so it just makes sense that we would use similar cues to remind us to think on more positive lines. You do this enough, and eventually, your mind will start to do it automatically, without thought or planning. Sometimes, we do this without noticing. For example, if you know you're going in to work with a very demanding boss, you mentally prepare yourself. You walk in with a spirit of wariness, and you've thought of everything you can think of to help you get through the day smoothly. You do the same if you plan to visit a sick friend. The same should also be true when you are preparing for a potential anxiety attack. The more you prepare your mind ahead of time, the easier it will be when you are actually working to push that anxiety back down to a level where it belongs.

Reject Your Inner Sensations:

Next, you want to recognize those negative thoughts and refuse to accept them. A gift is not a gift until you accept it. So, if your mind is flooded with negativity, realize that you have the option to say no to it. You are not compelled to accept any thought or feeling just because it came from your subconscious mind.

Our subconscious mind has been trained by our myriad of experiences that we go through from the moment of birth. Sadly, we have often forgotten the experiences that led to our negative thinking, and only the thoughts remain. Just as we said earlier in this book, change is a natural part of life, and any experience you had that shaped your negativity and fears most likely no longer exists. Learning to say no to such things will help you stabilize your mind and put you in a more positive perspective.

Find Your Safety Zone:

No matter how bad we think something may be or has the potential to be, it is always easier to handle when we know that we have a safe place to run to. Our safety zone doesn't always have to be a physical place to hide. It can be a form of meditation or just a mental state you train your mind to run to when things get to be too much.

Because of the crazy world we live in, most of us have forgotten how to live. We are constantly on the watch, focusing our attention on potential dangers, threats, malice, and pain. When we fall into that line of thinking, we feel everything is not safe. Start making it a habit to look for the good things in your life. They are there, hidden away behind a wealth of badness, but you can find them. You just have to look for them.

Change Your Inner Critic:

We all have that inner voice that is constantly reminding us of our past failures and our faults. This is not a characteristic exclusive to those with an anxiety disorder. It is common to all of us. But we have to start making a concerted effort to put that voice on mute. Those harsh words were drilled into us years ago, possibly when we were children and couldn't do everything right. But now, we have to change that dynamic. Up until this point, it has been a one-way conversation with that tiny voice buzzing all these negatives in your ear. It's time for you to start talking back to it.

Our inner critic acts like a judge that has nothing good to say. It judges the quality of our work, predicts how other people will view you, and makes you feel guilty and ashamed at every turn. It mocks you, teases you, and bullies you. He doesn't care about your feelings and has only one goal, and that is to prevent you from having any joy in life by questioning and doubting everything you do.

Identify the Judge:

One of the first things you need to do is identify your judge. If his voice is constantly ringing in your ear, the chances are that you are not even noticing it anymore, you are automatically responding to it without even being aware of its negative prodding. You'll notice when your judge is there when you finally get up enough nerve to tackle something, and suddenly your energy starts to wane, you begin to question yourself, or without reason, you lose interest. Recognize, at this point, that it is your judge, your inner critic who is taunting you.

Stop and listen to what he has to say, but don't respond to it. Don't resist his words because that will only build up the anxiety in you. Start a dialogue with him, refuting all of his arguments. For example:

Critic: "Why are you doing that? People will think you're strange."

You: "So what if you say that. It doesn't mean it's true."

Critic: "Do you really think that others will care

about what you do?"

You: "Who cares what other people think. Do you think I want to live with others judging me?"

Critic: "You're not going to be able to finish that, so why even bother."

You: "I'm doing this for me, not for someone else."

Whatever you hear, your inner critic tells you, don't remain silent. It's a tiny little voice in all of us. But the important thing is to acknowledge what he says, respond to it, and then keep moving on. That little voice inside our heads is there to serve as a warning to keep us from getting into danger. But there are times when he gets a little too much power and warns us even when there is no threat.

The inner critic rarely goes away. As long as we're living, he will continue to find ways to sabotage our efforts. However, if we can identify who he is, acknowledge that we've heard him, and forge on in spite of the fears he creates, his voice will not have as much power over us, and we won't have to worry about succumbing to our fears.

A Word at the Right Time

Another mystical tradition that has done wonders to help relieve anxiety is the use of affirmations. Because you're caught in a loop of negative thinking that has undoubtedly taken its toll. The use of positive affirmations is a great way to interrupt those negative thoughts with something positive verbally. It aids your mind to shift its thinking and gradually guides the mental process in another direction.

You can use these affirmations in three different ways.

- You can say them silently to yourself.
- You can write them down.
- You can say them out loud to yourself.

Anytime you feel overwhelmed with negative thoughts, and you can use these positive affirmations to redirect your thoughts in a more positive direction. Some therapists recommend that you make it a habit by attaching your affirmations to something you do every day. For example, every time you get in your car, you repeat your affirmations. Or you could say them every time you go to prepare a meal, put your children to bed, or hang up the phone. The trick here is to make it a regular habit to use these affirmations until they become a natural habit to you.

Some examples of positive affirmations you could make to fight off anxiety:

- I am calm.
- I am a good person.
- I value who I have become.
- I am healthy.
- I feel relaxed.
- I can let go of this stress.
- I am a good student.
- I can make a new friend today.
- I have a good relationship with my family and friends.

There are some basic rules about creating your own affirmations. First, all affirmations must be used in the present tense. Do not make mantras about the future or refer to something in the past. Second, they must always be about you. You are battling your own inner thinking process; therefore, your affirmation should be there to redirect your thinking. This is the only thing you have any control over. And third, they have to be 100% positive. Do not use any words like can't, don't, won't, etc. Instead of saying I can't get angry anymore, rephrase it to say, "I am going to stay calm today."

Many people question the value of something as simple as positive affirmations. However, while they are not an actual cure for an anxiety disorder, they are a powerful coping technique that will work for you until you can get the benefit of more long-term treatment options. You can think of them as a means to counteract those negative thoughts while you are working on something else. They are there to give your brain an alternative way of thinking.

While they are commonly used when negative feelings and thoughts pop up, some have found they do better if they start their day with affirmations, letting them start on a more positive note.

However, you choose to use them; they can help ease your anxiety in many ways:

•They are a positive distraction and can keep your thoughts from running wild.

•They give you a positive belief. In time, the brain

will adapt to the positive phrases and start to adapt to the belief that you are trying to form.

•And they serve as a constant reminder to insert more positive things in your life.

Make sure that the affirmations you choose have personal meaning to you. While you can find a long list of suggestions online, one that you create yourself will have more influence over your thinking than something written by a total stranger.

You need to be committed to using them regularly. It may take time before you begin to see the benefits, but if you continue, eventually, you'll start to feel the anxious discomfort fade away replaced by something more positive and actually makes you feel good.

CHAPTER 12
MAINTAINING POSITIVE MINDFULNESS

As you can imagine, embracing positivity in everyday life can make a profound change in how happy and peaceful your overall life is. When you utilize a positive mindset every day, you will find that life, in general, tends to flow and unfold with more ease and that people in your life then start to respond back to you in more optimistic ways.

I am sure you are aware of this, which is one of the main reasons you are here in the first place! But the real power is behind actually doing it, not just talking and reading about this positive picture. Trust me, I know the struggle of everyday life, and that it can be a lot to handle. Even during amazing experiences and opportunities, the chaos and demanding challenges of life seem to overshadow the greatness you do have.

While motivating yourself to maintain positivity every single day is not easy, it is more than possible and certainly worth the effort.

First, positive people are almost always positive, no matter what, because of two key things:

1. The practice being optimistic about strengthening this capability further.

2. They choose to be positive because it feels a heck of a lot better than drowning in a pool of negativity.

We are not born positive or negative, and one person is not more capable of optimism from the next. Stop making excuses about your skills, challenges, or situations you are enduring when it comes to your level of optimism. There are no aspects that make positivity easy, even though many see it this way.

Positivity is primarily a choice. You need both free will and awareness to succeed and maintain a good sense of optimism in your life. Guess what? Every person, even you, is wired with free will and conscious awareness! You are always in a good place to be more positive and start reaping the benefits from it.

When you are aware of yourself and your life, you will then notice when you are starting to venture down the path of negativity. Having this awareness jumpstarts the choice between optimism and pessimism. Below are some awesome tips you can begin to practice to gain optimum results!

Ways to Be Happier Daily

Practice the Power of Positive Thinking

The power behind positive thinking is undeniable. When you think positively:

- You receive better results. When you love the new evidence of improvement, you strive further to achieve it continuously

- You better notice your flow of behaviors and choices. You are better inclined since you know how you are feeling and thinking.

- You create better results, and others in your life respond in favor.

- You feel more at ease.

- You behave in a more optimistic manner, thanks to the elimination of the negative cloud raining over you daily.

- You have less time for negativity when embracing optimism.

- You allow your mind to be fueled with more positivity, which has amazing effects on your physical, mental, and emotional health.

- You are better able to recite positive statements to yourself.

- You actively choose to utilize the power of positive thinking each day.

When Faced With a Challenge, Choose Positive Responses

Problems are inevitable and will arise. It is just a part of life. We all face them, but it is critical to our overall wellbeing how we interact with issues. When you negatively react, you end up majorly draining your energy and affecting your health in bad ways.

Positively facing challenges at hand does not necessarily mean you are forced to be happy about them. It is about learning to choose the best perspective in all situations. We all have a choice of what type of perspective we choose, which, in return, affects how we feel.

Here are ways to embrace positivity no matter the scenario(s) you are faced with:

Instead of locking in your first negative thought, ask yourself these questions :

- What is the situation teaching me?
- What is a positive, more peaceful way I can interpret and approach this situation?
- Take a moment to breathe and count to 10 (sounds too simple but work wonders.)
- Take notice of how you are feeling and thinking.
- Realize that you have the ability to pick your perspective, and nothing can make you think anything. Remember that your mind is a sacred place that is yours.

Practice self-love

The bulk of all positivity and the greatness that comes with it begin with you. It has little to do with what is happening in your life and everything to do with whatever is happening within yourself. When you feel good about yourself, it is much easier to jump on the path of positivity.

If you don't believe or love yourself, you are bound to face numerous challenges when it comes to generating a positive attitude that is required for success in life.

To help create a better relationship with yourself, you need:

- to do something at least one time per week that is an act of self-care. Think about any action you take to make yourself feel nurtured and supported. Even think about things you do for others or that you do for those you deeply love and start doing similar things for yourself!

- to practice the art of forgiving yourself instead of beating yourself up about weaknesses, goals that are unmet, regret, mistakes, the past, or guilt.

- to take stock of the things you do love about yourself. Anything from skills, achievements, triumphs, strengths, etc. Learn to love the journey you have been on so far.

Daily Actionable Steps for Positivity

I became aware of the power that a positive, habitual routine played in my life once I honestly started to embrace and utilize it. Here a few things I personally use in my daily positivity routine, plus some others that people find helpful in their day-to-day lives to radiate optimism:

- Regular exercise.
- Planning out your day.
- Listening to uplifting music that plays a part in motivating and inspiring you.
- Praying or having a conscious conversation with life and the universe.
- Gratitude.
- Visualization practices.
- Meditation routines.
- Listening and speaking positive affirmations out loud.
- "Thought Interruption Technique".
- Jot down recurring negative thoughts.
- Write out an alternative thought for each one.

- When you are aware of negative thoughts, practice interrupting them and instead, recite the positive thought to take its place.

- Repeat those positive thoughts until it becomes familiar to you.

- Choose to end every day on a positive note so that you are able to capture quality sleep.

- Celebrate every achievement.

- Give thanks and learn to be blessed with what you do have in life.

- Repeat affirmations that help you feel better about yourself.

- Listen to guided meditations.

- Journal things that inspire you and motivate you to live a more positive lifestyle.

Ways to Have Happier Thoughts All Day, Every Day

If you learn the power of harnessing positive thinking, you are more likely to attract positive circumstances in life. The same goes for negativity. The more pessimistic you are, the more negative situations will arise. The blessings you receive in your life are ultimately up to you. If you think and act positively, you will then unknowingly call positive things to appear. If you are pessimistic and cynical, you will always be caught up in a whirlwind of negatively self-inflicted prophecies.

Like attracts like!

Meditation

I was skeptical about meditation at first, but once I started utilizing it in my everyday routine, that skepticism quickly faded. It has been one of the best and one of my favorite methods of removing negative emotions from my life and recovering with a nice dose of positive emotions and spirituality.

Meditation works to rejuvenate your mind, which makes it much more resilient when negativity does arise in your life. It not only rids us of all those bad chemicals, stress, and anxiety in a physical way but in an emotional sense as well.

I like to explain meditation to my readers like this: If you are always wired to be miserable, meditation should be viewed as a big RESET button that allows you to unplug, turn off, and tune out. Meditation is a practice that can be easily learned and implemented so that when you turn your brain back on, it is now using frequencies of positive thinking instead! Pretty cool, right?

If you use meditation often and long enough, you will discover that a lot of the damage that negativity has caused becomes eliminated, and you are left with a nice, clean slate to paint all on your own with your new positive mindset.

Be Thankful

Gratitude, no matter in what context, always has the power to instill more happiness in our lives. In fact, scientifically, it gives our brains a big dose of dopamine, which is a 'feel-good' chemical that erases negative emotions and thoughts.

Gratitude is an action that conjures the law of attraction we have discussed previously in this book. If you make an honest effort to be grateful, you will find that you end up being blessed with more! Make sure to write in that gratitude journal every single day. I like to do so right before I hit the hay. (That rhymed!)

Be Kind

Kindness is another proven action that washes the stress away and leaves us feeling joyful and content with our lives. Kindness is contagious within the human race. When a person is kind to you, you feel motivated and very inspired to pay it forward, right? That is how much power it holds!

Kindness is also an action that helps to influence gratitude as well since it makes us more inclined to be truly blessed.

Stress-Less

If only life were 'stress-less,' right? Since this will never be the case unless you live in a hole and never come out for sunshine, you need to learn how to extinguish the flames of stress and all of the unhealthy things that come with it such as anxiety, depression, and addiction, to just name a few.

Stress is caused by dwelling on the things that are going wrong in our life. Stress is often classified as 'emotional distress,' which, believe it or not, is self-inflicted. If you work too hard, you will start to become unhealthy. If you do not sleep enough, you will become exhausted. If you neglect your friends and family, you will develop loneliness. So, how does one win?

You must rid yourself of life's negativity and choose to relax. This means take care of yourself, both inside and out. Drink lots of water, eat right, exercise, meditate, get enough sleep, etc. Learn never to bite off more than you can consume. When you practice self-care, you will start to feel the stress fall away from you.

Be Your Biggest Fan

Tell yourself at least once per day how talented you are, how gorgeous you are, and that you are just plain AWESOME. When you do this every day and make it part of your routine, you will start to believe it truly. Pep talks work for folks. They uplift, inspire, and motivate you to make the best in your life every single day.

The next time your gut feeling informs you that something is wrong, instead of saying to yourself, "This is bad," affirm yourself that you can handle whatever life throws your way and tell yourself, "I will be okay."

Pulling Positivity from the Rubble

There will be times in your life that it feels like the entire world is against you even though you are doing everything to stay above water. It may be a reason why you are still reading this book. In chaotic situations, it can be difficult to remain positive, which may incline us to act out in negative ways. Well, you see what good that does, none. This will only attract more negativity to your life, and at the end of the day, no one wins this game.

If anything, negative situations are calling out in dire need for you to stay positive and ride out the tides of bad situations. There are ways to stay positive that I have learned to use, especially when it seems like life is crumbling around me.

Ways to Easily Optimize Positivity in Negative Situations

- Know that it is not possible to please everyone in your life. No one has the power to do this, no matter how hard they try. You need to realize that you will have to let certain people go throughout your life to relieve negative burdens.

- View negative situations you are in as "training sessions" that will help you to succeed later in life. The higher you climb, the worse situations you can get. These scenarios are preparing you for future endeavors.

- Have favorite motivational and/or inspiring quotes, either memorized where you can recite them to yourself or placed where you can easily see them every day.

- Talk to someone that is a positive influence in your life to help encourage you to keep trucking forward.

- Learn to admit to the mistakes you make openly. Remember, you are human, and no one in this world is perfect.

- *One of my favorite quotes to remember regarding mistakes:* "A life spent making mistakes is not only more honorable but more useful than a life spent doing nothing."

- Holding onto negative feelings and emotions will do more harm than good. There is no good reason for you to grasp pessimistic points of view.

- Learn to maintain a positive point of view of those in your life. Even if you do not like their behavior or the message they are sending, it doesn't mean you should hate them personally. This hate only makes you harbor dark negativity that is hard to shake.

- If you come across negativity in people or messages, learn to ignore and avoid them. They are a waste of your valuable time.

- What do people say about you? View the content in a positive light so that you can act upon it and improve yourself. Don't avoid and reject messages people are trying to get to you.

- Learn the power of speaking in a gentler tone to help reduce tension in situations.

- Take a nice, deep breath to calm yourself down when the going gets rough, so you are able to think clearer and in a more positive manner.

- Don't respond when you are angry. If you are not sure if you are calmed down, do not respond to something until you know you are.

The Five Rules of Positivity in Negative Situations

In situations that are hard to keep up a positive persona, it is even more essential to stay positive, so those around you do not judge you by your inability to handle situations that arise. Negativity only tends to make things worse, which later fill you with more resentment, anger, disappointment, and later guilt. No one has time for this.

The tried and true way to beat negative situations is to keep and maintain an optimistic attitude. This is a choice you must make, especially when seeing difficult scenarios as learning curves instead of a huge pothole in your road to success. Here are the five rules of staying positive when life gets hectic.

Rule 1: You are in control of how you respond

You and only you can control your response to situations. Take deep breaths, count to 10, and do whatever you can to remove yourself from the negativity that tries to overrule your behavior. When you are calm, you are more able to think clearly about how to solve things.

Responding in correspondence to how you are

feeling will only make the situation worse than it already is. "If you cannot say anything nice, then don't say anything at all." A good rule of thumb to adhere to!

Rule 2: Learn from negative situations

It is easier said than done, but viewing pessimistic scenarios as opportunities to grow and learn helps you to find opportunities in difficulty. Instead of using your energy to react negatively, do something positive to help make the situation at hand better.

Rule 3: Admit mistakes

As a society, we tend to forget that we are human and are allowed to make mistakes. We all have shortcomings. But one thing we can do to make situations better is to admit our mistakes instead of trying to deny them. Learn from the mistake you made that developed the bad situation, learn from it, and move forward.

Rule 4: Maintain a positive point of view

In negative situations, our opinions have a funny way of becoming jaded. This is when remaining positive is essential so that we do not allow ourselves to jump to conclusions. When you become proactive in dealing with the adversity of certain circumstances, you can help to affirm yourself and your positivity.

This is especially important when we are forced to work under pressure. It can be difficult to keep up a positive attitude, but this is where positivity plays a key role in developing a good or bad outcome from a situation.

Rule 5: Highlight the Positive

- Don't go back and forth between negative and positive emotions. When negativity comes to the surface of your mind, flip back to an optimistic point of view and remain there.

- Make the positive truths concrete by being true to yourself and your life's work.

- Discard all negative thoughts that are born from pessimistic situations. There is nothing good to be gained from acting out in a bad way.

- Affirm your attitude with your words and actions, not just one or the other.

-

Easy Ways to Live a More Positively Driven Life

To reduce anxiety, one must be willing to put in the work to make positive changes and better ways of thinking a habit. There are many small changes one can make that can potentially have significant positive results in their life. This chapter is full of just a few of the best ones!

Mindful Moving

We are a species that tends to live in the future. Everything we do in the present moment is aimed towards a potentially better outlook in the long run. We forget to take the time to enjoy and live in the present. When you spend more quality time at the moment, it is much easier to be positive and have realistic expectations. If you spend all your time in the future, you are just setting yourself up to be a major worry-wart. Move slowly during your morning routine, and the rest of your day will hopefully be followed by the same action.

Start Off Your Day Positively

The method in which you start off the day from the very beginning sets the tone for the remainder of it. This is why it's so often stressed to get up a bit earlier so you can perform your morning routine at your own pace. We often are functioning at full speed and are susceptible to getting lost in stress and the loss of power we have over our lives.

Add Value to another Life

The vibes we send out into the world daily have a funny way of coming back to hug us or kick us right in the butt. What you give is typically what you receive.

- **Help out** – Lend a hand to a friend when they need it, give someone a ride, or ask someone if they need assistance.

- **Listen** – Learn how to listen instead of talking over people. Most times, people just need a listening ear that is non-judging and attentive to what they are saying.

- **Boost moods** – Give hugs (when appropriate), smile at people while making eye contact. Play feel-good tunes when hanging out with friends or suggest an inspiring movie. Encourage those going through tough times.

-

Don't Let Fear Overrule Your Life

There will be times you want to take life by the horns, be risky, and take a chance. But anxiety has a way of pulling you back from these opportunities. We tend to spew out vague fears to make excuses for not taking chances. We are fueled by fear instead of what is possible if we try. Ask yourself what the worst that could happen is. This will make way into figuring out how to spend time in unfamiliar situations that could lead to potentially bigger turnarounds.

Find Your Happy Place

It turns out that finding your happy place is a real thing and is especially recommended for those that experience periods of anxiousness. Mentally relocating ourselves when our anxiousness flares up is a great way to remain relaxed, calm, and in the moment. It gives us the freedom to lose ourselves in a moment. Happiness is a state of mind. The more you practice getting there, the easier it will become for you.

- Recall places that you have been that you have liked for their sights or sounds.

- Use the method of imagery or visualization to bring about that place you seek.

- Ensure that you choose a place that you experience happy emotions.

- Try to recall where you were when those feelings of deep meaning and/or contentment engulfed you.

- Maintain open-mindedness.

Write

I know that writing has helped me time and time again when it comes to my feelings of anxiety. Whenever I was feeling particularly anxious or in some type of emotional turmoil, I would grab a notebook, my phone, or my laptop and jot out my feelings. To do this effectively, let go of your fear of judgment. Unless you give your journal or whatever you write on to someone else to read, this is just for you to vent. It also puts a positive spin on being an anxiety sufferer.

I have created many great reads, such as short stories and poems, from what I was feeling at a certain moment. Do not think of writing as attempting to avoid anxiety. You are living in that moment by not only documenting it but over thinking about it in a constructive manner. Seriously, try it. I assure you that you will feel much better about it. Plus, if you write often enough, you may see a pattern in your life that you wish to or need to change.

Find the Optimism within Negative Circumstances

I have found that one of the most effective ways to create a positive point of view on any kind of situation is to ask more helpful questions. What is good about the situation? What is a new opportunity that might be lying within it? Thinking like this has a much more positive effect on my life than asking what I did to deserve this, etc. Do not rush these inquiries, though. Take time to process your feelings and thoughts towards a situation. Trying to force positivity while in emotional turmoil usually isn't very effective.

Cultivate a Positive Environment

The more time you spend from outside media such as television, magazines, or the World Wide Web, the better. It is essential to have positive influences in your life to lead your life in such a way. Ask yourself what some negative influences in your life might be and what sources of information lead to negative thoughts. When going through your answers to these inquiries, think about how you could spend less time around these things. You now have a lot more time free to do things that will make positive impacts on your life!

Be Comfortable in Your Own Skin

This one can be a challenge, especially for those who suffer from anxiety. We fear judgment and try to be perfect when, in reality, no one on this planet can achieve perfectionism. Learn to accept who you are and the body in which you were born. If you constantly wish to change things about yourself that are impossible to change, you will never be happy with yourself. It kills any potential to be happy. When you are not comfortable in your own skin, this leads to problems with confidence, self-esteem, and overall well-being. Distance yourself from people who make you feel less than happy.

Appreciate What You Have

If you are always seeking for what others have and what you don't, you will always picture your life as the grass is greener in other people's yards and not appreciate and become grateful for all the wonderful things you have in your life already! You will constantly feel miserable and as if something is missing. This is the same for comparing yourself to others, as well. While it may set a certain benchmark to achieve success, comparing yourself with others does become unhealthy at some point.

Make sure your motives are aimed towards prosperity. Simply learn to appreciate what you have and take time to acknowledge that everyone is fighting their own battles. You would be surprised by just how many people wish they had your life.

Let Go of Anger and Resentment

Resentment towards other people is only going to poison you to the core. We hang on to anger with the assumption that the person will eventually realize what they did wrong. But, we are only hurting ourselves. Learn to let go and forgive, no matter how long the process takes.

Live with an Open Mind

Those who are narrow-minded are only hurting themselves. You will feel agitated more so than those that live openly because of how firmly you stand in beliefs that many others may not live by or approve of. If you learn to live your life as your own and respect that others are more than capable of living theirs as is, you will be happier overall.

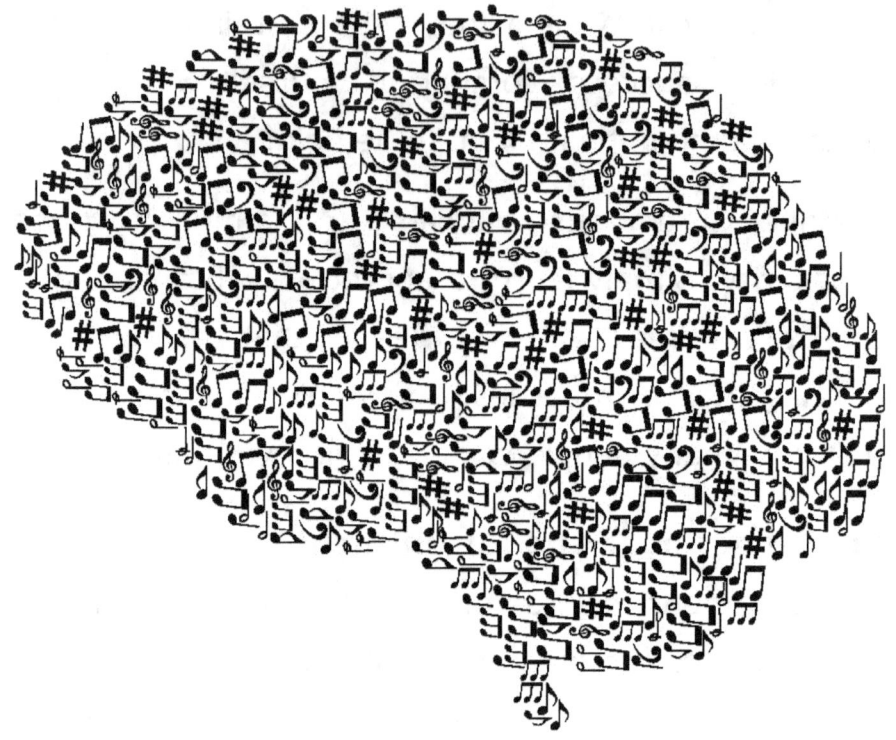

Listen to Music that Reflects the Mood that you wish to be in

There are plenty of studies to show what impact music has on our brains. If you want to be in an upbeat mood, turn up your positive music! It is a surefire way to brighten your day. Share it with those around you! I know, for me personally, getting out and driving for a bit with my music blared with some of my favorites, upbeat tunes help my anxiety out immensely.

Other Ways to Live More Positively

- Wake up with the strongly held belief that today will be a great day.
- Inform those that you love that you care about them and their well-being.
- Unhappy? Only you have the power to change your life.
- Things will not always be bad, tough, or rough. Things will get better.
- Make a list of the things going right in your life instead of dwelling on all the things going wrong.
- Engulf yourself in your favorite activity or hobby if you are stressed. Anything that boosts your mood is approved!
- Even when things do not go your way or happen unexpectedly, learn to view things as positive mishaps.
- Learn to be easy on yourself. Do not always strive for perfection.
- Enjoy nature or other places that help you escape from reality for a bit. This can be

soothing and help automatically relieve anxiety symptoms.

- Turn up your favorite song. It is a sure-fire and quick way to perk up!

- Balance your time wisely between work, school, relationships, and yourself.

- Each day is a gift. Treat it as such.

- Research has shown that those who are optimistic tend to live longer!

- Unplug and take breaks from social media, schoolwork, and workplace projects. <u>Everyone needs and deserves a break sometimes.</u>

- Eat things that nourish your body. A healthy vessel gives way for more positive energies to be felt throughout the day.

- What are you passionate about? Learn to become a master at whatever drives you.

- Adequate sleep, rest, food, and exercise all play roles in a healthy lifestyle and mind.

- Laugh often and smile as much as you can!

CONCLUSION

Getting through life with a mental illness isn't always easy, whether it is a major depressive disorder, general anxiety disorder, social anxiety disorder, obsessive-compulsive disorder, or any one of a number of other disorders. However, with cognitive-behavioral therapy, you can transform a painful and torturous life into a joyful and fulfilled life. No longer do you have to simply push through all of the negative emotions and experiences brought on through your disorder. Instead, you can transform your life with a few simple techniques and hard work.

Cognitive-behavioral therapy will take time, you can expect it to take twelve or more weeks to experience the full benefit, but it is well worth it. Studies have regularly shown that CBT is one of the most effective treatment options for both depression and anxiety, with the longest-lasting results. Medication is rarely enough on its own to control these disorders, but with the addition of CBT, you can keep your mental health in check and prevent relapses.

Before you began this book, you were likely unsure, afraid, and at your wit's end. Yet, you now have all the answers you need to regain your mental health and take control of your life. You can begin to enjoy life, smile, and laugh again, no longer having depressing and anxious thoughts control your every move. All you have to do is begin. Don't wait. Begin week one now, and in twelve short weeks, you will be in a better place. You can be happy again. You can feel like yourself again.

www.ingramcontent.com/pod-product-compliance
Lightning Source LLC
Chambersburg PA
CBHW071404210526
45465CB00001B/251